# Becoming a Medical Doctor: Is It the Right Career Choice for You?

# Becoming a Medical Doctor: Is It the Right Career Choice for You?

*Dr. Michael Clifford Fabian*

iUniverse, Inc.

New York  Bloomington  Shanghai

# Becoming a Medical Doctor: Is It the Right Career Choice for You?

iUniverse books may be ordered through booksellers or by contacting:

iUniverse
1663 Liberty Drive
Bloomington, IN 47403
www.iuniverse.com
1-800-Authors (1-800-288-4677)

Because of the dynamic nature of the Internet, any Web addresses
or links contained in this book may have changed
since publication and may no longer be valid.

The views expressed in this work are solely those of the author and do not necessarily reflect the views of the publisher, and the publisher hereby disclaims any responsibility for them.

ISBN: 978-0-595-45468-6 (pbk)
ISBN: 978-0-595-89780-3 (ebk)

Printed in the United States of America

# Contents

# *Acknowledgments*

I would like to thank Dr. Gary Bloomberg, Ms. Lisa Blum, Dr. Samantha Cogan, Ms. Angelina Desjarlais, Ms. Kim Katz, Dr. Michael Seear, Dr. Doron Sommer, Dr. Deborah Terespolsky, and Mr. Daniel Wulffhart for reading my manuscript and for their helpful comments.

# *Preface*

Are you considering applying to medical school? Have you wondered whether medicine is the right career for you? Choosing your career is one of the most important and difficult decisions you are likely to face, and struggling with such a crucial life decision is not uncommon. It may be your dream to become a medical doctor—it is a wonderful career with many exciting aspects—but it's no secret that the road to becoming a medical doctor is difficult. If you are uncertain whether you should follow this career path, or even if you are simply curious about the field of medicine, this book is for you—it offers answers on a broad range of topics.

As I look back on the past twenty years of my career, I can recall the excitement I encountered each step of the way—from the time I received my acceptance letter to medical school to the most recent phase of my career. Still, it's important to understand that the first step on your journey—the selection process for medical school acceptance—is quite competitive. The available spots in any medical program are reserved for high achievers. Even the application process itself is challenging. And after you have been accepted to medical school, the training and long hours involved are intense, and the stress level is high. The sacrifices you will need to make to pursue a career in medicine are enormous. So why place yourself on such an arduous and stressful path? Because a career as a medical doctor is extremely rewarding, with a level of job satisfaction that is hard to find.

This book will help you as you weigh the pros and cons of choosing medicine as a career. This is not a career you should choose lightly; as a potential medical student, you need to understand whether you and medicine are a good fit. This book also addresses the particulars of entering medical school, the options you'll have after becoming a medical doctor, and many other important factors associated with this career choice.

In this book I offer my insight, based on my years of medical experience—in medical training, medical practice, surgical practice, research, education, and my work as a medical admissions administrator, as well as my observations of others in the field. I offer a candid overview of the points to consider when contemplating a career in medicine.

The book is intended as a practical guide to help you decide if a career in medicine is right for you, and if so, how to pursue it. It also offers a look at the "big picture" while focusing on the fine details. For me, this profession has been an enlightening and rewarding experience, which I would like to share with you. I hope you will enjoy reading this book as much I enjoyed writing it.

# *Introduction*

There are many amazing aspects to the medical profession. There are also some aspects that are less than amazing. As a potential medical doctor, it's important to take into account all the positives and negatives associated with this choice. I have devoted much of this book to discussing the positive and negative reasons for choosing medicine as a career. The one resounding concept you should take away from this reading is that to have a successful career in medicine, you need to have an unconditional desire to help others. Helping people is a large part of why many doctors love being doctors. In the pages to come, I will introduce and discuss the BOAT concept. This acronym stands for the unconditional desire to help a person despite his or her **b**ackground, **o**utcome, or level of **a**ppreciation, and with disregard to the **t**reats (or secondary gains) you, as the doctor, may obtain. If you can honestly embrace the BOAT concept, you most likely have made the right decision about becoming a doctor.

Your career aspirations, however, may have been dependent on your stage in life. As a child, you might have been asked, "What do you want to be when you grow up?" Of course, the choice you made then may have been without a true understanding of the secondary implications of a career choice—financial remuneration, lifestyle, and social status. As a child, you simply named the career of your dreams.

As you matured, your career choices may have swung from one extreme to another—or you may have known from a young age that you wanted to be a medical doctor. Regardless of whether you have always known that medicine is the career path for you, or you have recently come to this decision, it's important to recognize that you need a strong desire to succeed and a will to endure whatever it takes to reach your goal. Most important, however, you need to honestly enjoy the process. While it is essential to have clear and specific reasons for pursuing a career in medicine, it's also valuable to acknowledge that there are wrong reasons for embarking on this journey.

I cannot stress this strongly enough: Being well suited to the medical field is of paramount importance. It is vital to recognize whether or not you have the necessary personality traits and characteristics to succeed in the profession. There is no magic formula to determine who should go into medicine, of course, but I hope that this book will provide helpful insight.

I find it interesting to observe doctors who are following their dreams via their own unique path. The way I see it, there are two potential roads that lead to a career in medicine: the *fast track* or the *alternate track*. Those who are on the fast track generally have made up their minds early in life that they want to become physicians. They apply to medical school as soon as they meet the requirements, and they likely have taken college courses geared toward fulfilling the standard requirements for some medical schools. Taking premed courses allows them to maximize their knowledge, which places them in the best-possible position to be accepted into medical schools that require such a background. Many medical schools favor a science background, but institutions do exist that favor other backgrounds, such as humanities, so it's wise not to limit course choices to those that seem exclusively designed for future application into medical school. This concept is covered in more detail later in this book.

The alternate track describes the road taken by those whose medical school plans have been delayed. Some might be undecided about their career choice, and they may prefer to obtain a general degree while contemplating their future plans. Others might want to experience different aspects of life—such as taking a year off to travel—before embarking on an intense and expensive university program. (This is often a wise choice, as it becomes increasingly difficult to take time off after beginning medical school.) Some might have a financial situation that precludes them from entering medical school. The aspiring medical student then must work and save money before embarking on a university experience. And some simply have personal or social situations that prevent them from entering medical school until later in life, for example, personal or family health problems, personal relationship issues, or the desire to start a family. Other reasons are covered in more detail later in this book.

Some people may ultimately choose other health-care careers, such as a career in osteopathic medicine, naturopathic medicine, podiatry, chiropractic, dental surgery, nursing, midwifery, optometry, occupational therapy, physiotherapy, or pharmacy. There is a lot of interaction between medical doctors and these allied health-care professions. In many ways, the goals sought by pursuing a career as a medical doctor can be equally achieved by pursuing a career in one of these related fields. These alternate choices are covered in more detail in the chapter titled "Other Career Choices Related to Medicine."

Gaining knowledge of and exposure to the medical field is paramount to making an informed decision to apply to medical school. But due to the current privacy and confidentiality laws with regard to medical information, it has become more difficult to gain access to patients in a clinical setting. Patients also may be uncomfortable with having you sit in on their doctor visit. This book will cover ways in which you can get much-needed contact and exposure to the medical field.

The years you'll spend in medical school and in subsequent specialty training are exciting, but these years also are intense—this is something you need to fully understand. Having prior knowledge of all the factors associated with this time will help you to make an informed career choice. In this book, I attempt to explain what medical school and post–medical school training are actually like—the good parts as well as those that are less favorable—with frank discussions and a synopsis of the multitude of specialty choices.

This career continues to be unique, as opportunities continue to expand for practicing physicians. This array of diverse options includes clinical medicine, academia, research, administration, pharmaceutical involvement, policy making, and business endeavors. Additionally, clinicians can choose a particular type of practice with which to be involved, and physicians can choose to run a solo practice, be a part of a large teaching hospital, or a number of other options. These different opportunities are covered in detail in this book.

Many aspects of the medical field change over time: screening methods, methods of diagnosis, medications, surgical treatments, and alternative medicines. As a physician, you'll need to keep up with advances in health care and stay on top of changes in your chosen field—it's your personal responsibility to remain up-to-date, but it's also a requirement of the governing and licensing bodies. This continuing learning process, however, is a major attraction for many who choose to become medical doctors.

Other factors to consider when choosing a career in medicine also will be covered in this book, for example, licensing, mobility, technology, innovation, challenges, audits, and litigation. These factors aren't necessarily foremost in your mind when you've thought about becoming a doctor, but it's beneficial to cover all aspects of the profession—this is the big picture.

Ethical considerations in the medical profession also are important, yet they're often misunderstood. You may hear the term "professionalism" (as it relates to ethical behavior) repeatedly throughout medical school. The concept is very much a gray area, and many universities are actively reviewing the standards and expectations relating to professionalism. Personally, I like Merriam-Webster's definition: "the conduct, aims, or qualities that characterize or mark a profession or a professional person." Many of the basic principles relating to ethics are covered in the text of the Hippocratic oath; the modern version of that oath is discussed later in the book.

During the course of this book, I will provide examples that demonstrate certain points or concepts. I also will share experiences from my many years in the medical field, offering personal experiences from family practice, pediatric practice, surgical practice, research, education, and administration. In this way, I hope to illustrate how wonderful this career path can be.

My intent with this book is to clarify the different aspects of a medical career as you consider medical school, and I hope to help you make an informed decision. I further hope that my efforts will contribute to a generation of healthy and happy physicians, who genuinely enjoy their profession. If you enter the field of medicine with your eyes wide open, it can be extremely rewarding.

# 1

# *The Right Reasons for Choosing Medicine*

A career in medicine will allow you to improve the lives of your fellow human beings through modern medical care. This dynamic field has continual advancements, requiring you, as a physician, to keep up-to-date in whatever medical discipline you choose. This ongoing learning process will keep your curiosity piqued, even as it provides you with new knowledge and information. I know of many physicians who have continued to contribute to medical education and volunteer within the medical field even after they had retired, which attests to their passion for the medical field.

People who are attracted to a career in the medical profession generally possess specific attributes, the most basic of which is a desire to help people. A career in medicine offers many different paths, such as clinical work, research, education, or administrative interests, and it further expands into a multitude of interests or specialties. Some areas of medicine can be procedurally oriented, while others can be laboratory based. All the different aspects of this career allow medical students a certain degree of liberty in deciding which area of medicine they would like to pursue. Still, I feel that it cannot be emphasized enough that the most important reason to become a doctor is because you have an unconditional desire to help people.

After becoming informed about your career choice, it's important to adopt realistic goals and expectations about the field of medicine. If you, as a potential student, are aware of and understand the important reasons for entering the field, your motivation will be much clearer and stronger. Situations are likely to arise after you become a physician that may cause you to question whether you made the right career choice, but if you are able to reflect back to the factors that were taken into account when you decided to become a physician, your ambivalence is more likely to be resolved.

In considering my own unconditional desire to help people, I devised the acronym BOAT to help you understand my sentiments in this regard. I have an unconditional desire to help people, notwithstanding the following four things: the **b**ackground of the patient; the patient's **o**utcome; the **a**ppreciation level of the patient; or the **t**reats (secondary gains) that may come my way.

I believe the BOAT concept is a fundamental concept to consider before choosing a career in medicine.

## B is for background.

A person's background may include age, gender, race, religion, educational level, profession, socioeconomic status, sexual orientation, marital status, political beliefs, native language, physical disabilities, and physical appearance.

At times, a patient's background characteristics will conflict with your values and expectations. In these situations, you are expected to detach from your personal beliefs and values, and treat the patient as any other. Certain levels of accepted practice and standards of care define how a physician should make decisions and treat patients. While personal beliefs may be at the forefront in the decision-making processes of other areas, a doctor does not have that liberty. Doctors have to do what is right for the patient in a system where the codes of ethics and practice are clear. As a doctor, holding to your personal opinions could present a challenge for the patient, the medical institution, and yourself. For example, abortion is permitted in certain health-care facilities, but some physicians refuse to perform the procedure. If you are a physician who has a moral disagreement with performing abortion, it is your responsibility to recommend another doctor to your patient; thus you provide care for the patient while not performing the controversial procedure yourself.

Consider the following real-life examples where background factors came into play:

**Example 1:** Homeless people often present an unclear medical history, making it difficult for the physician to assess and treat them. Homeless patients are sometimes unable to verbalize their condition or symptoms; they may become verbally abusive or combative; they are often in poor physical condition; and they may not have access to bathing facilities. It is common for these patients to have an accompanying mental illness. Some patients, not just the homeless, might be infected with transmittable diseases, such as HIV and hepatitis B or C.

As a medical student or physician, you may not yet have experience in dealing with patients from a variety of different backgrounds. When you made your decision to enter medical school, you might not have considered that tending to homeless or mentally ill patients was part of the job description. But as a physician, you must be willing to provide medical services, regardless of the patient's condition or background. Sometimes, administering care may require that a patient be physically restrained or sedated; this forced care can be quite traumatic for the healthcare providers, and tough decisions frequently have to be carried out on the spur of the moment. If you are a doctor in an emergency room setting, you could be dealing with such situations on a daily basis, yet the patient's background should not determine the level of care he or she receives.

For your own protection, you must adhere to blood and body fluid precautions when dealing with any patients—particularly when dealing with patients who are suspected of or are known to be infected with transmittable diseases but also with patients who show no signs of infection. Most medical schools and residencies require that at least a portion of a doctor's training take place in an inner-city hospital, facility, or office. Therefore, exposure to this population group cannot be avoided.

Further, some doctors choose to work in an inner-city hospital, where the most disadvantaged patients turn for care because, while challenging, this aspect of medicine can be particularly rewarding as patients are helped on the road to recovery.

**Example 2:** Communication problems can result if patients do not speak English, and there may not be an interpreter readily available. Performing a comprehensive clinical assessment and providing the best-possible medical care can be very challenging when a language barrier exists. Such a situation, however, can be part of your daily life as a physician, and you must willingly help all patients to the best of your ability. In large medical institutions, there is usually at least one person on staff who will be able to speak the patient's language. If not, however, you must do your best to determine the patient's complaint. You might, for example, use hand signals, or point to specific parts on your own body and look for confirmation from the patient to determine if the patient is experiencing pain in a certain area.

You may set up practice in an area where a particular ethnic group resides, where the majority of the patients do not speak English. I found myself in this situation, and I considered it an opportunity to learn a new language. While practicing as a surgeon, I worked in an area largely populated by Italians. Most of my patients were seniors who had come to North America from Italy at a later stage in life, and many were unable to speak English. I learned basic Italian, mostly words and phrases that related to the office environment and that were of a medical context. It gave me much pleasure to converse with my patients in Italian, albeit a broken dialect on my part. In addition, the patients respected and appreciated the fact that I made an attempt to speak their language.

**Example 3:** A person's lifestyle may be directly against your beliefs and values as a doctor. For instance, you may be caring for a homosexual patient who has decided to start a family. In such a situation, your patient may seek your support and advice on how to move forward. Your own background, comfort level, personal views, and religious beliefs can pose a major dilemma in controversial situations, but it is your responsibility to put these aside in such situations. Treat all patients on an equal footing, despite any personal conflicts you may have. The bottom line is that patients rely on you to provide them with care and often to provide care for their family members too. The support you provide as a doctor will usually be appreciated, regardless of the patient's personal situation. Being on the receiving end of that appreciation can make for a good day at the office. It will help you remember why the field was so appealing in the first place.

## O is for outcome.

Doctors want everything to go well for their patients, but there are times when contributing factors—those beyond a doctor's control—will influence a patient's outcome in an unfavorable way. Patients and family members will have high expectations of you, and with those expectations comes the misconstrued notion that you, as the physician, will be able to save and cure their loved ones. Some medical conditions, however, are incurable, despite having access to the most advanced medical treatments available. These include some cancers, chronic medical conditions, mental disturbances, and life-threatening injuries, among many others. With disorders of this nature, patients may have an unfavorable outcome regardless of your medical care. But in such instances, you still can experience a sense of accomplishment by helping a patient through a very difficult situation.

As a doctor, you must be prepared for the certainty that at some point, regardless of how you work to save a patient's life, his or her death may be unavoidable. And it is important to know that some areas of medicine have a higher likelihood than others that a patient's outcome will be negative or fatal. Examples of these fields include specialties such as oncology (treating incurable cancer being a common part of this specialty), cardiology (heart attacks and abnormal heartbeats are two examples), and some surgical specialties, such as cardiac surgery and neurosurgery. Keep in mind that these fields can also be the most rewarding, because there is little else in life that can match the act of saving someone's life.

Having spent many years in a pediatric environment, I know that there is little worse in life than seeing a critically ill child. Here, I offer two real-life examples.

> **Example 1:** A young patient was being looked after by his grandparents while the boy's parents were out of the country. The trio was spending the day at a cottage on a lake, and the grandparents lost sight of the child. In that short time, the boy had managed to jump into the water and wasn't found until a few minutes later. After being rushed to an area hospital, the boy was placed in the intensive care unit (ICU); he was critically ill and on life support. Hospital staff then had to contact his parents to tell them what had happened. In this situation, there were three tragic events to contend with. First, there was a dying child in the ICU; second, the traveling parents had to rush back from out of the country to face the horrific situation; and third, the grandparents were devastated and had the burden of guilt on their shoulders. As the child's situation became terminal, both the parents and medical staff had to increasingly support the grandparents, who were gravely affected by the tragedy. The child was deemed brain-dead and was eventually taken off life support. It was a very difficult time. Everyone, including the staff, shed tears, and I will forever carry vivid memories of the situation. This child's death was certainly not an outcome that I could have predicted when choosing a career in medicine and a subsequent specialty in pediatrics. But despite everything, this experience had a positive side in that everyone involved—family and hospital staff—leaned on each other and supported each other through this tragic event.

> **Example 2:** While I was working as a family doctor, one of my elderly patients developed a rare type of blood cancer. There were no cures available for this condition, and it was just a question of

time as to when he would die. I became very involved with his terminal care and was supportive of the family during this difficult time. Clearly, I had no control in terms of saving this patient's life, but I felt that I was helping the situation in many other ways, particularly by lending support to the family. When my patient died, the family was not angry that I couldn't save their loved one; they expressed their appreciation for all I had done for him throughout his last days.

Undesirable outcomes are simply a fact of being in the medical profession; at some point, they will be unavoidable. Yet these experiences can make for a rewarding career in another way—by helping patients and their family members through the dying process. Doctors who choose to specialize in areas where positive patient outcomes occur less frequently may choose oncology or palliative-care medicine.

## A is for appreciation.

We all like to be appreciated for what we do, but it seems as though being unappreciated is prevalent in the medical field. This may be because people in the medical field often deal with life-or-death situations, and not all family members are appreciative of care that ends with a loved one's death. They may lash out against doctors, nurses, and medical students. After a loved one dies, the family or friends of the deceased often give no thought to thanking the medical staff that aided them. Even when the outcome is positive, family members, friends, or even the patient himself may not express appreciation for your efforts. For this reason, it's important to reflect on the principles that led you to a career in medicine in the first place—likely, it wasn't to receive someone's thanks. Focus instead on the enormous amount of personal gratification you receive from saving or improving the quality of life for an individual. Consider the following examples:

**Example 1:** When I was working as a surgeon, I was to perform a procedure on a child who had been having tonsil problems for many years—many infections and severe breathing problems that resulted in the decision to remove the tonsils. Prior to taking the child into the operating room, I met with her parents. Because their concern had been apparent during preoperative visits, I knew that they were very worried about their daughter's well-being. On this day, however, their concern seemed focused on whether I had filled out the insurance forms so they would be compensated for the time they'd taken off work to attend the surgery and assist their child after surgery. (I appreciated their high stress levels at that time and made every effort not to judge them for their actions.) The surgery was not an easy procedure, due to scarring from previous tonsil infections and resultant bleeding. Despite the challenging nature of the operation, how-ever, I was happy to report to the parents after surgery that their child had done well and was waking up in the recovery room.

But instead of offering their thanks, the parents seemed more con-cerned about other particulars—who would check on the child before discharge; who would be available by phone if there was a problem; when would the child's prescription be ready. While these were relevant concerns, I had expected that the parents might express relief that their child's surgery had gone well and without complications—and that they might praise me and show apprecia-tion for the successful surgery. The nature of their questions clearly demonstrated that the parents cared for their child's well-being, yet they expressed no appreciation. In this instance—and in many others like it—I had to put things in perspective and realize that the parents were stressed and focusing only on what to do next. My spirits remained high because I knew that I had helped this young patient by performing the best-possible surgery that I could.

**Example 2:** During my time as a surgeon, I once was urgently asked to come to the emergency room while on call as the ear, nose, and throat doctor. I jumped out of bed in the middle of the night and drove to the hospital as quickly as I could. Upon arrival, I encountered a young adult male who was gasping for air. His throat was severely swollen—he had a neck infection—and his skin had a bluish hue. I could tell that the situation was rapidly deteriorating; patients in this clinical state can die before your eyes. The emergency room staff had exhausted all its options, and the staff members were anxiously awaiting my arrival. I rushed the patient to the operating room, and a staff member called the patient's mother to inform her of the situation. For an ear, nose, and throat surgeon, this is one of the most difficult and high-risk situations that can be encountered—an airway needed to be obtained immediately. This required me to perform a tracheotomy (incising the neck to bypass the airway obstruction) and insert a breathing tube into the trachea (the man's breathing passage). There are a lot of important structures in this area of the body, including large blood vessels that supply the brain. In addition, in this situation, there was no time to administer anesthesia—that means that the patient was awake for this procedure. This patient was also confused and combative due to oxygen deprivation and had to be restrained so that he would not move.

I managed to get that breathing tube safely in place, without a major hemorrhage and in time to save the patient's life. Also very exciting to me, though, was the prospect of being able to tell the family that I had saved their son's life.

But instead of expressing appreciation for this happy news, the family barraged me with questions: "What exactly caused this? Why wasn't it picked up earlier? How long is he going to be in the hospital?" There was not a thank-you to be heard. I had rushed to the hospital in the middle of the night and dealt with a highly stressful situation, even though I faced a busy day at the office within a few hours. Again, it was important for me to reflect on the situation and realize that I'd saved the young man's life. Even though the family did not express appreciation, I knew that I had done my best—and saved a life.

Sometimes, thanks come later, after the acute stage has passed; sometimes not. I have come to realize, however, that the act of helping someone in distress is one of the main reasons I decided to pursue a career in medicine. The appreciation of the patient or his family should not be an issue.

## T is for treats.

One of the things you may hear from fellow medical students is that they one day hope to have a Porsche, a big mansion, or an exotic lifestyle. Acquiring these "treats" is not a good reason for pursuing a career in medicine; status should never be a major motivator. Be a doctor because you want to help people, save lives, and improve the quality of life; don't choose this profession because it will bring you financial treats. There are numerous other, often easier, avenues to achieve financial success. This area is going to be discussed further in detail in the next chapter.

There are many other valid reasons for choosing a career in medicine. While you know your own reasons, there does seem to be a common thread among most prospective medical students.

Among the major benefits of a career in medicine are choice and flexibility. As a doctor, you will have many options once your basic medical training has been completed, and you must decide whether you want to pursue a family practice or one of the many specialties or subspecialties available. Many people prefer being generalists, while others choose to specialize in a clearly defined area. If you choose to become a specialist, you then can choose whether to subspecialize in a particular area. The spectrum of specialties is vast and continues to expand. This allows you to narrow down your choice of specialty or subspecialty very finely. You also must decide if you will concentrate on clinical medicine, academic medicine, research, education, administration, or a combination of these. (For more information on available opportunities after obtaining your medical degree, see chapter 6.)

Past experience can be a positive motivating factor for going into medicine. Some individuals consider medical school after experiencing a medical problem themselves or witnessing one in a family member or friend. These students are likely to enter the profession with a desire to make a change, perhaps stimulated by a situation where lack of knowledge about a condition or disorder led to an unfortunate outcome. Remember that medicine is a dynamic and ever-evolving field. You may choose to enter medicine in the hope of finding a cure for a particular condition or to develop technology that may improve or save people's lives. Part of the joy of pursuing a career in medicine is the realization that although we have come very far in understanding the human body, we still have a lot to learn about disease onset, detection, diagnosis, and treatment. The desire to make a specific change is not an unreasonable motive for pursuing your dream of becoming a medical doctor, but it must be combined with other factors.

> **Example:** One of my colleagues entered medicine later in life because he wanted to make a specific change. While my colleague was working in another health-care field, one of his children faced a life-threatening illness. As a result of the anguish and sorrow my colleague endured, his desire to help people, and because there was no cure for his child's disease, he was stimulated to pursue a career in medicine. He hoped to help other children with the same disease to live better and longer lives. Not only did he complete his medical schooling, but he also completed specialty training and ultimately became a pediatrician. He is now able to help many sick children, including those who have disorders similar to the one his child had, and he is doing a great job at it. The sense of accomplishment in that type of a situation is enormous on many levels.

Conducting research might motivate some to pursue a career in medicine, and research is definitely needed for medical advancement. Taking the time and making the effort to go to medical school is a long road to travel if you are planning to pursue a research-based career. Attending medical school and training as a resident, however are essential steps that must be taken if you wish to be a clinician-scientist. Keep in mind that although many schools look at research as a positive characteristic when selecting their medical students, the weight given to research on a medical school application differs from one institution to the next.

Financial stability often comes into play when making a career decision. Although this should not be a primary focus when deciding if you should go to medical school, it is certainly an important factor, and it must be considered. The medical field in most parts of the world has reasonable financial remuneration and job security. In fact, physicians often fall into a higher income bracket than most other occupations. In some geographic locations, a physician is able to decide if he or she wishes to practice as a solo physician, in a group practice, or in a hospital setting. In some areas, the physician is also allowed to decide if he or she would rather work on a salaried basis or provide services on a fee-for-service basis. (In some countries, fee-for-service is referred to as private practice.) Many physicians choose to combine two or more of the above-mentioned alternatives. For example, a doctor may choose to balance a solo practice with a part-time academic appointment that could involve teaching and research. Also, combining two or more areas of medicine might provide better compensation, if one area pays less than another. While the pay is generally good for physicians, keep in mind that becoming a physician often requires a large financial catch-up period because most doctors have accumulated a large amount of debt by the time they graduate from medical school and complete their residency. In North America, the term "residency" is used to describe the additional time spent in training to achieve competency in the area of medicine of your choice. This is, however, a relatively high-paying field, and paying off of the loan might not be a burden for too long.

Job availability and job security are usually excellent. Some specialty positions are more difficult to obtain if you have your heart set on a specific location. This is because some locations are saturated with doctors of a specific specialization. There always will be a job available somewhere, but securing that job may require relocation. Job availability and security becomes more difficult when moving to a different state, province, or country. Unlike other careers, in the medical world, it is very rare to lose one's job once a position or practice is secured.

Unemployment is not usually a problem for medical doctors, but this statement is applicable to those who have not trained in a province or country of residence but who are citizens or permanent residents of that jurisdiction. An example of this might be if you presently live in Canada but did training in Asia or South America. You would be considered for-eign-trained, and as such, you'd lack the appropriate training and licensing requirements for Canada. If this were your situation, you'd have no choice other than to choose an alternate career or go through additional training. Many foreign-trained doctors, however, are able to practice in a jurisdic-tion other than where they trained; this depends on many factors. One factor is physician demand. It is not uncommon for governments, state legislators, or provincial legislators to ease up on restrictions imposed on foreign-trained doctors if there is a significant shortage of doctors in a par-ticular region. The practice of medicine might be restricted in terms of visas, duration, and location, but it is common for foreign-trained physi-cians to be recruited to rural or underserviced areas within a province, state, or country.

In general, a medical career has the advantage of being fairly mobile. There is often reciprocity relating to training and certifications among provinces, states, and some countries, but often there are requirements of further examinations and sometimes additional training before doctors may practice in a region other than the one in which they were initially trained.

You may choose to study at an institution far from your hometown for medical school, residency, fellowship, or even a sabbatical. This may be due to the prestige of an institution or the expertise of its instructors. Or you may simply want to move away from your home environment, albeit temporarily, for the required training. Remember, though, that you may not be allowed to reside in a different country after your training period due to visa or immigration limitations. Also, there is no guarantee that your home country will accept you as a doctor if your training was done elsewhere. While mobility is a good thing, it is imperative to research all factors involved before choosing training in a specific location, particularly out of the country.

It is also important to note that policies change. What may be in place when you begin your training may change by the time you have completed it. There may also be potential issues if you choose to leave your home country to study medicine in a foreign country. Often, this move is driven by the inability to obtain a training position in your institution of choice in your home country. The competition for positions is incredibly fierce, and too often, competent and qualified applicants do not get a desired spot in a local or regional medical school. In North America, it is not uncommon for someone to move to Australia, Ireland, or the Caribbean to study medicine when his or her original plans for studying in North America don't work out. Rules for licensing change continuously, but there is usually a way to return to your home country to work as a doctor at a later time. The options, however, for those who are not accepted at an institution in North America are to either study medicine in a foreign country or to not study medicine at all. To my mind, if you are drawn to study medicine, it is worth it to leave your own country for the opportunity to study, especially when the alternative is choosing an entirely different career.

The decision to pursue medicine as a career should be well thought-out, and all options should be considered. As a prospective medical student, you should ultimately make the choice to apply to medical school based on good reasons and motives and avoid using the wrong reasons as a driving force. As was illustrated in this chapter, there are many good reasons to pursue a medical career.

# 2

# *The Wrong Reasons for Choosing Medicine*

As with any career, if you choose medicine for the wrong reasons, it will make for a very unhappy work existence. The importance of job satisfaction cannot be underestimated. During your working years, you will spend a lot of time at your job. It just makes good sense to choose a job that makes you happy. Bad career decisions not only affect your well-being, but they also impact your personal life and the lives of those around you.

One of the most common "wrong" reasons for choosing medicine as a career path is for the monetary gain. Pursuing a career as a medical doctor based on the money you hope to make is one of the biggest reasons doctors become unhappy with their career choice. There is no question that being a physician leads to a stable career with a reasonable income and significant material gains, but this does not—and should not—compensate for job satisfaction. This is not to say that financial achievement isn't important, but it's more important to choose a career that will make you happy.

Some doctors feel trapped in their careers. After spending ten to fifteen years training to get where they are, they finally realize that their career choice is making them unhappy. While there is no guarantee that you ultimately will enjoy your chosen profession, you should be very certain you are choosing medicine for the right reasons. Of course, anyone can change the direction of his or her career, but often, once people have financial obligations and are settled in with a spouse or partner and family, it's not as easy to give up what is already established in order to make a change. Additionally, there may be other things to consider, such as a mortgage, private school tuition, or other comforts that are often associated with wealth. These considerations limit the doctor's ability to change direction, relocate, and pursue a new career path, even if he or she is unhappy. There is nothing worse than being trapped in a situation with no way out, especially if the situation was avoidable in the first place. Choose wisely the first time.

If you choose a career in medicine for the social status, keep in mind that the novelty of being a physician usually wears off. Social prestige is not a good trade-off for a career that makes you unhappy. I recently commented on this point to a friend who is not a physician, and she reminded me that regardless of a person's job, there will always be some aspect of it that is considered less than desirable. It's important to keep this in mind. Job satisfaction is all about balance; if you dislike more things about your job than you like, then the job becomes a problem. When the desire for elevated social status is relied on as the main driving force in a doctor's pursuit of a medical career, he may ultimately decide that he does not love what he is doing.

I must admit, though, early in my career, I wasn't immune to enjoying the status of being a doctor. Like many medical students, one of the most exciting moments of my journey was when I was first walked around with a stethoscope around my neck. I took advantage of any opportunity to give that stethoscope some exposure. But although the stethoscope started off prominently displayed around my neck, as time passed it was relocated to my pocket; it then moved to the briefcase. Later in my career, the stethoscope was nowhere to be seen. The "status" of wearing it was not nearly as important after decades of being in the medical profession as it was when I first began my career. I hope you can realize this fact as you start along your career path. Social status is transitory and not a good reason for choosing the medical profession.

You might think that if you truly loved your medical career, you would always want that stethoscope around your neck. Wearing a pager has much the same "status" for some young doctors—they see it as a way to impress people with their importance. And you might think that your pride in wearing a stethoscope or a pager is simply a reflection of the joy and passion you have for your chosen career. To a certain extent, this may be true. But as with any profession, the initial excitement of beginning your new career will dissipate over time, and that's when you will realize that there is more to being a doctor than the social status it brings. The job is more than walking around with a stethoscope around your neck or a pager hanging from your belt. It is crucial to be fully informed about all aspects of your chosen career prior to making such an important life decision.

Another "wrong" reason for choosing medicine as a career is to give in to external pressure. Parents and other family members may have encouraged you to pursue a career in medicine, and the expectation that you will follow this path can be ingrained from a very young age. If so, you may be under an enormous amount of pressure to follow through and become a doctor. Getting into medical school might be your smallest hurdle; surviving medical school, residency, and medical practice will be the major challenges. Using someone else's expectations as your driving force is a very bad decision. You need to have your own strong desire to become a doctor.

Having one or more family members working in the medical field is another reason some people choose a medical career, and that may work both as an advantage and a disadvantage. On one hand, you may have been exposed to the life of a physician, which may have created a deep understanding of what it is like to be a doctor. You likely have overheard telephone discussions with hospital staff and colleagues, and this could provide insight to the challenges and problems that you might face. Also, you might have witnessed firsthand the enormous satisfaction that can be obtained by helping people and saving lives. You also will have seen how much time the career involves, and you will know how to weigh that time commitment when making a decision about pursuing a medical career. On the other hand, having members of the family in the medical field might impose that expectation that you should follow the same path. Or, if your family member has been unhappy with his or her own career choice, he or she might have tried to discourage you from applying to medical school. It makes me unhappy when I hear a physician say, "I will never let my child go to medical school," or "I've discouraged my child from choosing medicine as a career." This is not uncommon, however, and it demonstrates how unhappy those people are with their own choice to become a doctor.

One factor that is worth mentioning is how the media, partially mainstream television, has expanded significantly when it comes to the variety of programs and shows relating to medicine. They can range from the documentaries that are quite informative and graphic to soap operas and comedy shows, which may or may not be a true reflection of medical training and practice. One thing is for certain; if you are concerned about your ability to tolerate the gory aspect of medicine, watching documentaries about surgery that include detailed accounts of the procedures might seal your decision either way!

You may consider medicine to be a glamorous field. Everyone will look up to you when you're a physician; you will be able to meet the partner of your dreams because you are a doctor; you will be invited to all the important functions in town; you will have lots of money—the list goes on. While these things aren't entirely untrue, the "glamour" wears off during the day-to-day challenges you'll encounter as a physician. This exciting career will be truly appreciated only if it is chosen for the right reasons.

# 3

# *Are You Suited to the Medical Profession?*

Once you decide to pursue a career in the medical profession—based on valid reasons and being well-informed—your next question should be: "Does my personality fit that of a medical doctor?" There is no right or wrong personality; medical doctors have a vast array of personalities. Just look at any medical school class, physician group, hospital staff, medical society membership, or alumni society membership; physicians' personalities span from one end of the spectrum to the other in terms of temperament, communication skills, sensitivity, arrogance, and patience. In medicine, people usually associate different personalities with specific areas of specialty. Pediatricians are stereotypically thought of as more caring and soft-spoken, and less arrogant; surgeons are often considered more aggressive, less patient, and somewhat arrogant. Of course, a stereotype is absolutely no guideline, however, it does you give you some idea as to how people can think when it comes to different specialties.

In order to determine if you are well suited to the medical profession, consider that vocational guidance counselors, psychologists, and therapists can conduct comprehensive testing and analyses to determine what professions are best suited for the individual. It would be to your benefit to seek out one of these professionals for an analysis of your probable suitability to be a doctor, based only on your personality. However, this type of testing may make generalizations that are not valid for every individual.

A few of the areas that I see as valuable in helping you understand if you're suited to the practice of medicine are as follows:

## Have a reasonable ability to retain information.

You'll need this to get through medical school, a residency, and practice as a physician. If you have reached the application process and have the grades needed to get into medical school, you already have displayed that your memory is good, that your ability to retain information is not a problem. Medical school requires that a large volume of work be covered in a short period of time. This intense period of training really tests the memory. Depending on your educational background, this may be more work than you have ever been asked to comprehend and retain at one time. As a young medical student, it was a big adjustment for me to learn to cover this large volume of study material in so short a period of time. But it's not just while you're in medical school that retaining information is important. Let me give you an example: During my days working as a surgeon, an elderly man collapsed and became unconscious during an assessment at my office. Although I had not dealt with this type of problem in quite some time, I had to quickly recall my previous experiences of a critically ill patient from my medical school days in order to intervene with this patient. There is a sequence of events that takes place in a situation like this, and often you'll have to rely on your memory to help the patient. You have no time to look in books, browse the Internet, or phone a colleague.

## Have the ability to process and comprehend information.

This is a problem for some individuals when the clinical years of training begin. Sometimes a student earns high marks through high school and postsecondary training, as well as in the earlier years of medical school and then suddenly starts failing clinical courses when the less-structured learning begins. There can be many reasons for this, but a likely one is the change in the style of teaching and learning that comes with clinical medicine. Transferring previously learned information into the clinical setting requires a very different way of thinking. This particularly comes into play when problem-based techniques are used. With support, remediation, and time, a person can usually resolve these processing problems. I recall one student who was a real star during his time as an undergrad and in the early years of medical school. Then, for some reason, once the problem-based learning and clinical medicine portion of the curriculum started, his marks dropped dramatically. He did not appear to be suffering from any personal or health problems that could account for this abrupt change. Eventually, after much help and support, the student continued successfully in the program, and his stumbling was chalked up to a change in the style of learning and knowledge application.

## Have a caring nature.

This is paramount to the daily life of a doctor. It is caring people who are attracted to medicine in the first place. During medical school, specialty training, and when in practice, you will repeatedly hear or make reference to "taking care of patients." This phrase is used daily in the life of a doctor, but we do not often stop to ponder its origins. In my opinion, the word "care" goes hand in hand with being a medical doctor. Warmth, sympathy, and compassion can be grouped together with the caring nature required of those who choose the medical profession.

## Have good interpersonal skills.

Such skills are essential. First and foremost, a doctor has to be able to communicate well with patients. During medical school training, residency, and while in practice, there is also ongoing communication and interaction with colleagues, staff, associates, trainees, and others. Not only are these interpersonal and communication skills important for the above interactions, but they also are utilized as an evaluation tool when being assessed in the clinical years. Performing poorly in this category is taken seriously by evaluators. No matter which field of medicine you choose, the course will be rocky if you do not have the ability to communicate and interact with people. While there are some areas in medicine such as radiology, laboratory medicine, or pathology that require little or no patient interaction, the ability to interact with colleagues and other staff is still of significant importance.

You've probably heard the term "bedside manner." Having a good bedside manner requires a combination of the personality traits mentioned above such as having a caring nature and good interpersonal skills. It does not matter how smart you are, how competent a physician you aspire to be, or how much you love your job. What is important to most patients is a doctor's bedside manner.

## Have patience.

Your patients want an opportunity to express themselves; they want to feel that you are listening to them. Some people are impatient by nature, including doctors, but it is important that you learn when to sit back and listen. There is also a fine line between being a good listener and knowing when to intervene and redirect the conversation toward pertinent information. Time is often limited; as a doctor, you must develop the skill of extracting the most important information from a patient within a brief time frame. You also must manage to collect important information from your patients without coming across as impatient or disinterested. There is no question that much of the medical world is money driven; that often means that doctors are expected to see as many patients as possible in the least amount of time, and this rushing through patients can contribute to doctors' job dissatisfaction. It's your job, then, to sensitively yet efficiently treat each patient.

## Be sensitive and empathetic.

Sensitivity is particularly relevant in the practice of medicine, but there needs to be balance. You must be sensitive to a patient's feelings and needs, as well as sympathetic to the patient's family, but you can't allow yourself to be so sensitive that you cry when something bad happens to a patient. Doctors do occasionally shed a tear, as do staff members and patients; this is normal. But you must remain strong and concentrate on the medical management of your patients; you must be sensitive but without becoming overly involved emotionally. Certain areas of medicine may be more emotionally challenging for sensitive individuals. As a future doctor, you will soon learn which areas of medicine are best suited for you. For example, during my pediatric residency training, I worked in the pediatric intensive care unit. While I enjoyed this time immensely, I found it very hard to be around critically ill babies. Pediatric intensive care is a subspecialty of pediatrics, and some doctors spend their entire careers tending to these children. Helping these very sick babies to get healthy can be an incredibly rewarding experience, but some of these patients do not survive. Those times are heartbreaking. Despite these setbacks, you must carry out the special care without becoming overly involved with every child and family.

## Have a strong stomach.

Some individuals would like to go to medical school, but they are squeamish and do not like the sight of blood. Your medical training requires courses and rotations in subjects such as anatomy, emergency medicine, and surgery. This education will not allow you to avoid the gory side of medicine. If you're unsure whether or not you're too squeamish, try to get some exposure to the medical field before making a decision about medical school. Consider volunteering in a hospital setting or an environment where you will see more of the blood and less of the glamour associated with medicine. Such exposure is critical; it is a vital step in helping you establish whether or not you can tolerate the "blood and guts" that goes along with training for a career in medicine. Even the strongest of individuals—those who have no reservations about going into medicine—can have a weak moment during medical school or specialty training. It is not uncommon to see a student or resident faint or express signs of dizziness following exposure to certain aspects of medicine.

During my early medical school days, a fellow medical student became pale, sweaty, and ultimately fainted while dissecting a cadaver. Cadavers are dissected from head to toe; this can be difficult for many students. I also crossed paths with many medical students and residents who felt weak or faint during my days working as a surgeon. The procedure that seemed to cause the most stress was a rhinoplasty—a nose job. During this procedure a surgeon literally uses a chisel and hammer to fracture bones for size reduction, correction of deformity, or resetting of the nose. The sound that the bones make as they crack and crunch may cause even the most experienced medical professional to cringe. Unappealing smells, in addition to sights and sounds, with procedures such as cauterization, can also be unpleasant for some individuals. And in case you're wondering, don't assume that women students are weaker in this respect than men—the men get weak and pass out just like the women do, maybe even more often! Even experienced doctors can experience a weak moment when witnessing something out of his or her comfort zone. An occasional fainting episode, particularly one that is related to a medical situation, should not preclude an individual from considering medicine as a career, but your ability to remain composed at the sight, smell, and sound of surgery, or aspects of medical care, should be taken into account.

## Recognize that death is unavoidable.

No matter what area of medicine you choose, at some point in your career, you are likely to have to confront death. Most medical students and doctors remember the first time one of their patients died. Seeing a patient die in front of your eyes will probably be one of your most vivid memories; you will always recall it clearly, even in your later years. No matter how prepared you may think you are for a patient's death, the first experience can be devastating. And depending on the field of medicine you choose, death may be a frequent event. You need to quickly learn to adjust to this fact of life and deal with these situations in the best way you can. Some doctors have a fear of their patients dying; this is quite normal and should not deter you from becoming a medical doctor.

## Be a professional.

Professionalism is a big part of being a medical student and a physician. In fact, it starts long before medical school, with the application process, when honesty and accuracy is fundamental. There are so many factors that relate to professionalism in the medical context, it is difficult to mention everything. Arriving on time to lectures, ward rounds, office visits, and the operating room all play a part in being a professional. Appropriate dress and language is also important when dealing with patients and their families. Cheating on your exams or copying other people's writings is obviously something that cannot be tolerated. There are many unprofessional things that can occur while practicing too, including changing previous patient notes, discarding important information, and lying to a patient. Reading the Hippocratic oath, which is included later in the book, will give you some insight into longstanding beliefs as to what professionalism entails.

## Be Ready to Give Up Some Of Your Spare Time.

Applying to medical school, attending medical school, taking part in post–medical school training, and practicing medicine can be very time-consuming and stressful. You have to make a sacrifice in order to pursue the career of your dreams. For those of you who have taken some time off to do other things, it will involve a significant change in mind-set and commitment in order to successfully complete your studies and training. Either way, a lot of spare time will have to be sacrificed to help pass those exams and get through medical school. I can certainly remember many a Saturday night when I had to stay home and study while some of my other friends who were not in medical school were out having fun. It is of the utmost importance that you are fully prepared for and understand the sacrifice that comes with becoming and working as a doctor.

There is no clear-cut personality type that is ideal for a medical doctor, but clearly there are characteristics that are compatible with the profession, just as there are personality traits that would make it hard for you to complete medical school or practice in many fields of medicine. The majority of those who go into medicine, however, have accurately determined that they are meant to be doctors—and they never look back.

# 4

## *How Do You Get There?*

There are many ways to achieve your dream of getting into medical school and becoming a doctor, yet there is no right or wrong way; each route has its own advantages and disadvantages. It is a competitive process, however, so you must be a high achiever at all levels in order to obtain that coveted spot in your chosen medical school. Successful applicants not only earn excellent grades, but they also maintain a balanced lifestyle and have other interests in life—the arts, research, leadership, sports, recreation, volunteering. Each person's journey is unique. The one thing I always tell aspiring medical students is that they must do whatever they enjoy doing to enhance their nonacademic portfolio. There is no sense in suffering through things in life that you dislike, just for the sake of getting into medical school. Fulfill the minimum required elements set by the relevant school, and after that, it is up to you to fill the rest of your life with activities that you find enjoyable.

There are two ways to get into medical school—on the fast track or on the alternate track. I define the fast track as getting into medical school in the quickest possible manner. If you're on the fast track, you will have made a definite decision about pursuing a career in medicine from a fairly early age. You may have known for as long as you can remember that you want to become a doctor. If so, an academic path can be molded as soon as practically and physically possible—it's a path that will culminate with your acceptance into medical school. There are, however, people who fit in this category but who cannot take the fast track to medical school. Despite knowing from a young age that they want a career in medicine, inability to obtain sufficient grades, personal reasons, or lack of support or finances prohibits them from taking the fast track. People in this group will have to put their applications on hold and take the alternate track.

For those on the fast track, it's always good to research the applicable medical school requirements to see how to structure your curriculum choices during high school and college. It is prudent to concentrate on subjects that focus on scientific knowledge in preparation for application and entry into medical school.

Most medical schools in North America still list the basic sciences as mandatory requirements. Basic prerequisites may include subjects like biology, chemistry, biochemistry, physics, and English. Humanities and social sciences are stressed at many schools as well, thus demonstrating how philosophies can differ from one school to the next. While you may have a plan for tackling the prerequisites, there is no guarantee that by the time your application is considered, the rules regarding prerequisites will still be the same. This is why I cannot emphasize enough that while a future medical student must prepare for acceptance into medical school, there is no point in designing your entire premed existence around essential studies and nonacademic activities that you do not enjoy. I strongly recommend that you read the information on the official Web sites of the Association of American Medical Colleges (AAMC), the Liaison Committee on Medical Education (LCME), and the Association of Faculties of Medicine in Canada (AFMC) for tips on structuring your studies and extracurricular activities.

Also for those on the fast track, it is vital to inquire as early as possible about additional exams or credentials that might be required for med school. As one example, the Medical College Admission Test (MCAT) is a prerequisite to the application process for most North American programs. The MCAT is a standardized, multiple-choice exam designed to assess an individual's problem-solving skills, critical-thinking skills, writing skills, and knowledge of science concepts and principles relevant to the study of medicine. Scores are divided into four categories: verbal reasoning, physical sciences, a writing sample, and biological sciences. The rules pertaining to this exam change periodically with respect to locations where the exam can be taken, the number of times the exam can be taken, and how long it takes to get the results. In addition, each medical school has its own set of rules pertaining to the MCAT. One school may require a minimum MCAT score, while another may limit the number of times a student can take the exam.

As of 2007, the MCAT examination has essentially gone paperless; computer-based examination centers have been set up across North America. It is important to revisit the MCAT Web site often to review updates. Many students find this a challenging exam, particularly if they have not recently completed any basic science courses. Books and study courses are available to help you prepare for the exam, but unfortunately, the study courses can be quite costly and thus not a possibility for everyone. If you truly want to pursue a medical career, however, these challenges should not deter you from moving forward. If you are on the fast track, consider taking the MCAT soon after completing the basic science prerequisite courses.

It is vital to gain some exposure to the medical field, even if you are positive you want to be a doctor. Ideally, you should get your first exposure while still in high school; there are often programs that allow a student to spend time with a physician or in a hospital. Additionally, many hospitals have volunteer opportunities available to students. This is a great way to gain exposure to the medical field and the hospital setting. Getting a job in a medical office would also be an excellent way to see what it's like to be a doctor. Besides gaining exposure to the medical field, this job would provide beneficial experience that could be added to your application when applying to medical school. As a prospective medical school applicant, it's important to be aware of building appropriate experience for an application to medical school.

Many options are available for those who are unable to pursue the fast-track route to medical school, that is, those on the alternate track. Many people see the alternate track as an advantage, but whatever your reason for delaying your application to medical school, this route allows you a longer period of time to decide if you've made the right choice and to gain some life experience. Many medical schools go out of their way to encourage mature applicants with qualities that a younger, fast-track student might not have been able to provide. Be aware of this factor when researching the institutions.

Many factors can be addressed while you are on the alternate track, such as indecision, suboptimal grades, previously being turned down for admission to medical school, financial instability, settling a desire to travel, or simply taking a break. High school and college can be stressful and intense periods in anyone's life. There is absolutely nothing wrong with taking a year off after high school or college to travel and work. Such opportunities will be more difficult to acquire once a medical career has begun.

If you have chosen the alternate track, follow the ideas mentioned in the previous paragraph in order to confirm that you have made the correct choice to pursue a career in medicine; having this additional experience might also enhance your chance of being accepted to medical school.

Students entering medical school later in life may not have experienced much exposure to the medical field. It may not have been possible due to other commitments, such as family or work. If you can arrange it, though, try to find a way to get some exposure to the medical profession prior to medical school. This is just as important for alternate-track students as it is for those on the fast track.

Use the extra time while you're on the alternate track to improve your grades, expand your credits, write qualifying exams (the MCAT being an example), or enhance the nonacademic experience. The advantage of this longer route is that you might be able to complete your prerequisite requirements without being pressured to finish within a limited time frame. This time can also be used to complete graduate work, such as a master's degree or a PhD program. You might complete these degrees as a planned sequence of events, or you might simply be in this situation because you weren't accepted to medical school the first or even the second time around. Graduate work, however, will serve as an alternative career option, should the application to medical school be unsuccessful. Some medical schools welcome and encourage academic or research backgrounds. Having a PhD gives the bearer a significant advantage over other applicants in terms of acceptance into their medical school. People often end up on a career path that was not initially planned—I know several people who initially planned to pursue a career in medicine until they found great satisfaction in their graduate work. Education is never wasted.

Remember, too, that the military can be involved with medical education and medical careers. You may be someone who is already enrolled in the military and have decided to pursue a career in medicine. The military might offer funding throughout your medical education, with the proviso that medical service to the military will be given once you are qualified. Or you might be someone who has joined a branch of the service at the beginning of your medical schooling so that the military will offer funding throughout your medical and specialty training. In return, after graduation, you will be expected to provide medical service to the military for a stipulated length of time. Working in the military can be exciting because you are able to serve your fellow human beings on many levels: health care, protection, and security for the country. Part of military work can also be humanitarian in nature, for example, distributing food and medical supplies. If you have interest in the military route, contact a military recruiter for more information.

Once you have decided that you would like to become a medical doctor, you must decide whether you want to pursue a straight medical degree (MD), a combined MD/PhD degree, or some other combined degree. By far the majority of people who are training to become a doctor are enrolled in an MD stand-alone degree and not a combined degree. For those who are interested in a research career combined with medicine, many universities offer an MD/PhD program. This takes longer than regular medical school training. In North America, the MD/PhD program takes approximately seven years. This would be of particular interest and an exciting opportunity for individuals interested in being physician scientists. The program is tailored in such a way that it affords you the ability to complete your PhD and fulfill the required elements for the MD portion of the training. There is usually a fair amount of latitude concerning the area of research the program might entail. For the most part, students in the MD/PhD program usually have been involved with some type of research prior to entering the program. The core medical training is the same as the regular MD route, and you will obtain the same clinical degree. There is no obligation on your part to pursue a research-based career, and you can decide later to practice in any field of medicine, provided your relevant residency training has been completed. Some universities also provide combined programs from disciplines such as basic sciences, business, administration, computer science, education, law, and public health. Every medical program's application and selection processes differ for these combined programs. Graduate research degrees may also be obtained during residency or fellowship training. Options available to you in combination with the MD degree are often not clearly apparent, so it is really important to explore the Web sites in detail and make sure you have covered all the possibilities available to you.

When you have made up your mind to apply to medical school, and if your situation allows for it, I strongly encourage you to visit the institution you would like to apply to, in order to make sure that it is a good fit for you. Aside from the educational aspect, you have to ensure that the geographic environment is in keeping with your comfort zone and lifestyle. There is no point in adding other stressors to a strenuous academic program.

No matter which route you follow, consider the benefits gained by having a mentor. A mentor in the medical field who can be an advisor and a pillar of support is always advantageous for the new medical student. A mentor also can be of high value when it comes to career counseling. He or she can help you decide whether medicine is a good fit for you. Mentors often continue their support throughout your time in medical school, specialty training, and well into your career. Most medical schools will have a program in place that can help you to locate a mentor.

So which is the preferred route—the fast track or the alternate track? Each individual must make that decision for himself or herself. My feeling, however, is that if you have made up your mind early in life to become a doctor, and you have the means to get into medical school, the fast track is best. But if there is any uncertainty about medicine as a career, or if there are other factors that make the fast-track route impossible, then the alternate track is the best choice. Only you can decide.

# 5

## *Preparing to Apply to Medical School*

Making the decision to become a medical doctor may be difficult, but the application process and capturing that coveted spot may be even more challenging. Once the decision has been made to pursue a career in medicine, you must place yourself in the best-possible position to get accepted, and plan the application carefully, because the competition to get into medical school is fierce. Let me give you some concrete examples of how difficult it can be. The Association of American Medical Colleges (AAMC) Web site publishes extensive and very helpful information relating to medical school admissions (http://www.aamc.org). For the entering class in 2007, at Harvard there were 6,642 applications for a class of 165; for Oklahoma, there were 1,288 applications for a class of 164; for Stanford there were 6,457 applications for a class of 86, and for Hawaii-Burns there were 1,901 applications for a class of 62. There are so many other good statistics on this Web site that can be very helpful when trying to understand the process and decision on a choice of school.

Academic achievement is not the only criterion that medical schools take into account when deciding which applicant to admit—it is crucial, but most medical schools welcome a broad nonacademic background. This can include such factors as employment experience, sports involvement, volunteer work, leadership qualities, research, publications, travel, and other life experiences. It's hard to gauge the importance of these extracurricular activities because they are weighed differently at each institution. The more evidence you show on your résumé that demonstrates your commitment to becoming a medical doctor, the better your chances are of getting into that program. These and other factors, including interviews, are important in determining whether you are worthy competition for one of the coveted spots.

It is crucial to research the university program and medical school to which you intend to apply. Universities generally offer details regarding the type of individual they are looking to admit. It is important to match yourself and your strengths with the best-suited program. Start looking for this information on a university Web site under the general policies, goals, and mission statements of the institution. The medical program usually offers some sort of elaboration on the type of individual they are seeking to admit to their program. The admissions section of a university's Web site should offer detailed information relating to the admissions process. The school may even offer the information in such a way that you can see statistics of the applicant pool and the accepted pool. Statistical information that may be available includes the average age of students enrolled, acceptance rates, average grades, minimum grades, gender distribution, educational background of students, geographic origin of students, and number of open spots available. The university might also provide the average accepted grade point average (GPA) and prerequisite courses. Some schools may go as far as offering the formula that they use to determine who gets an interview and how they make the final selection.

Other factors for you to consider when choosing a university are class size and the emphasis of the program as it relates to the types of jobs offered to its graduates. Some schools have large classes and a less-individualized learning environment. Others have significantly smaller admission numbers and class sizes. If you are most likely to excel in an intimate teaching environment, then this is an additional factor for you to consider when choosing the school you'd like to attend. Some universities or programs concentrate more on producing primary care or family physicians, while others will have a higher percentage of the graduating class going into academics, research, or specialty training. Once again, the Internet is a very useful tool for gaining such information. You can easily research different sources to learn medical school ratings. The *U.S. News and World Report* Web site even divides its rankings into two subcategories—the top medical schools in the United States that are research based, and the top medical schools in the United States that are primary care oriented. The Web site uses indicators such as acceptance rate, GPAs, MCAT scores, research grants, and ratio of students to teachers in order to grade the schools. While these tools are helpful in revealing the big picture, they should not be used in isolation for making such an important decision.

Also try to determine whether applying to a private medical school might be in your best interest. Private schools are able to function as a result of tuition fees and endowments, but the high personal cost may exclude you from following this road. The dream and commitment of going to medical school can be so intense that you may look at all options in order to gain admittance to a medical school, even if this means incurring major debt. In certain countries, such as Canada, funding is subsidized significantly by the government to cover the training of medical students.

Application requirements can differ immensely from one medical school to the next. Among those differences may be prerequisite guidelines, minimum MCAT scores, and minimum GPAs. Some schools might consider the GPA of all postsecondary courses taken, while other schools may use more recent courses or an average of grades received in all prerequisite courses. For those medical schools that require course prerequisites, there are differences in which courses are required. For medical schools where English is the first language, it is not uncommon for a school to require an English course to prove fluency, comprehension, and understanding of both the written and spoken word. In North America, the MCAT also screens for this. Be sure to familiarize yourself with all these details prior to choosing a university, choosing a program, and filling out the application.

Many schools have specific numbers with regard to how many applicants they will accept from out of state, out of province, or out of country; some universities do not accept out-of-country residents. It's a good idea to check for additional information on the programs and initiatives of a specific institution. For example, in Canada, some universities have specific programs in place to encourage and support aboriginal applicants who show interest and promise for pursuing a career in medicine. As another example, some countries have quotas in place in order to ensure adequate admission of qualified people from minority groups. Make sure you find out about this information from the relevant medical school.

Optimizing diversity in a medical program is a very current initiative in North America. It is important to ensure that the accepted class does not exclude any particular background in a community. For example, some schools have initiatives in place to attract and support individuals from a lower socioeconomic background. Unfortunately, many people are disadvantaged due to lack of opportunity or cultural background. A common criticism in many medical schools is the fact that the class is largely comprised of students from a privileged background. Making a medical class more inclusive of the local population in a geographic region is an area where much improvement is needed. It is particularly important to have doctors from all the different circles of life, including doctors of various races and socioeconomic backgrounds.

If you have a medical condition or physical disability, research the specific institution to which you would like to apply, with regard to its limitations. The mission statements of most universities outline that they encourage applicants with disabilities, and most indicate that they can accommodate students who are physically challenged, but let the school's technical standards guide you as to whether pursing a medical career at that institution is a viable option.

If you still have questions after consulting a university's Web site or the school's information package, contact the institution directly. Questions that are not admissions related might be redirected to another department, such as Student Affairs. This is a supportive and resourceful department for aspiring medical students. Some medical schools offer tours or an open house of the facilities for prospective applicants. Not uncommonly, there is a structured program in place to introduce prospective applicants or individuals already in the applicant pool to the medical school and university. Another source of helpful information is a premed or medical student society—this is a good way to get a clear view of the medical school from a student's perspective. These student body groups often organize educational programs that address the many issues related to applying to medical school and beyond.

Many medical schools offer advisory services for prospective (or rejected) applicants. These advisory opportunities may be provided at different stages during the application cycle, for example, before applying, after not being granted an interview, or after final selection. The quality and quantity of advisory services differ across the board. Some schools are against offering advice to rejected applicants; others feel strongly that providing any feedback is a valuable tool that may help an applicant to be accepted the next time.

Many schools like to see volunteer experience on application forms. Universities often outline how much volunteering they consider to be ideal and in what areas they like to see volunteer work, although most are flexible on this. If possible, start by volunteering at a health-care-related facility. Hospitals, nursing homes, and clinics often have organized volunteering services. In addition to looking good on your résumé, volunteering is good experience that offers personal gratification. You don't have to volunteer in a third-world country for your volunteering to be of value. Engaging in a humanitarian act on a local or regional level is just as beneficial in demonstrating your commitment to helping others.

It is also a good idea to have research and publication experience. Research can be performed at any stage of the academic process. Clinicians may welcome volunteers to work on research projects. Even if you are not in a full-time undergraduate or graduate research program, it still is beneficial to be involved in some type of research and, if at all possible, to have your results published.

Applications to medical school go through a cycle. The first part of the cycle is the deadline you must meet with regard to submitting your application. Complete your application thoroughly and well in advance of the deadline. Many institutions allow prospective students to apply online, where you also have the ability to log in and monitor your application's progress. If your application is submitted online at the last minute, however, you run the risk of the Web site being overloaded. Universities are not required to make concessions for this inconvenience, so don't risk it.

Apply early, whether you mail your application or submit it online. Transcripts and additional supporting information need to be forwarded well in advance as well—you don't want your application to be disqualified due to missing documentation.

Be accurate with your application. Misleading information can be picked up during the file review or at any other time the application is being considered for admission. Contact information is requested by some medical schools, and it is not uncommon for file reviewers to contact the applicant or the applicant's contact person to clarify details such as the number of hours spent with a certain activity. Don't make up facts to "impress" the admissions board. Dishonesty will undoubtedly disqualify you from moving forward in the application process and can possibly affect you in the future. Honesty and accuracy are crucial.

Most medical schools require an essay or personal statement of some sort to be completed as part of the application process. While you may be tempted to ask for help, especially if you doubt your grammatical skills, do not ask someone else to write this essay for you. This type of cheating is so common that it is easily picked up by the institution in different ways. If nothing else, the interview process is a perfect way to judge if a student's conversation matches the tone of the written essay. Honesty and high ethical standards are of utmost importance here—it really is a do-it-yourself project.

While it is important to be as complete as possible, do not unnecessarily pad your application with insignificant experience or achievements. The reviewers and interviewers want to see candidates who are being themselves.

The fees paid for applying to medical school can vary immensely from one university to the next. There can also be additional fees for those applicants who live out of province, out of state, or out of country. Additionally, many schools require a deposit to ensure that the applicant is serious about accepting an offer to that particular medical school. Just like the application fees, the amount of the deposit can vary from one school to the next. Remember, though, such fees and deposits should be considered a life investment.

Once submitted, your files undergo a review process. Depending on the university, this can be done in several ways. Sometimes, external individuals are involved in reading the files; at other times, faculty members, admission committee members, or members of the admissions team do the reading. Each institution has its own method of selection, but usually the files are narrowed down to a short list, and these people are granted interviews. The process for narrowing the applicants with regard to their files is another step that varies widely from one institution to the next. Some schools use the MCAT score alone for the first round of eliminations; other schools use factors such as GPA, prerequisites, and nonacademic qualities.

The interview process may follow different models. It may be a one-on-one experience, a panel interview, or multiple interviews with a number of different interviewers. Panels can consist of two, three, or more members. The university may build a well-rounded panel, including members such as clinicians, academics, community members, and medical students. These panel interviews can be structured, semistructured, or unstructured. Representation from different geographic areas within the medical school's recruitment area might also be taken into account when choosing panel members. These panel interviews may range from thirty minutes to an hour in duration. A relatively new interview model is multiple mini-interviews, which was developed by the Faculty of Medicine at McMaster University in Ontario, Canada. These mini-interviews put the candidate through a series of short interviews, one after another. These short interviews are usually about ten minutes long and consist of between eight and twelve stations. The idea here is that multiple assessments from a number of different people provide a more structured and broad assessment of the candidates' strengths and weaknesses. The content of the stations can vary from basic questions to scenarios, actors, collaboration, writing, or audiovisual stations. This method of interviewing has become increasingly popular with MD programs in Canada and globally. It is also being adopted as an admissions interview tool by allied health fields worldwide. Universities are usually transparent about how their interviews are structured, and they often provide feedback as to how the applicant performed.

Once the interviews are completed, the schools have different methods to determine the final selection of medical students. These methods can consist of formulas that take into account different aspects of your history and interview performance. Many schools, certainly those in North America, have committees that review your files in detail and vote as a group as to who finally gains acceptance to their program.

Receiving that acceptance note, e-mail, letter, or telephone call is something you will always remember. While the preparation for medical school and the application process can be difficult and time-consuming, when you get accepted, the time and effort will be well worth it.

# 6

# *What Is Medical School Like?*

Once you are accepted into medical school, you may experience a significant sense of accomplishment, relief, and excitement. The next few years, however, will be full of hard work as you study to become a medical doctor. Most medical school programs in North America last four years. Some universities do offer a three-year program, while others might be longer, incorporating premedical years within the curriculum. There are already two programs in Canada that are only three years long. In other countries, such as the United Kingdom, Australia, New Zealand, and South Africa, students have the option of applying to medical school directly from high school, thus completing a lengthy training program that includes the premedical training during the earlier years of medical school, followed by the clinical years. The duration of this route of training is usually five or six years.

Each university has its own curriculum, with most institutions covering the basic science-related aspects of medicine in the earlier years and the clinical training at a later stage. It is not uncommon to incorporate limited clinical skills and experience as early as the first year of training. Medical schools usually have a very structured curriculum. There are, however, stipulations handed down from accrediting bodies to make sure that core knowledge and basic procedures are included. Each year of training is divided into different blocks or rotations. There are also opportunities for students to choose blocks of time to experience areas of medicine that are of specific interest to the student. These are commonly referred to as electives or selectives. This time may be spent at a medical office or local institution, but some students choose an institution in a different city or even a different country. There is usually flexibility as to the nature of the elective. As an example, if you are interested in dermatology, you may arrange to spend a month with a dermatologist. There, you would gain additional knowledge and experience in skin disorders; you would have an opportunity to confirm a preexisting interest in the field; and you would have an opportunity to establish contact with a person who could serve as a mentor or a reference, should you decide to seek a residency position in dermatology.

Each university and medical school has its regulations with regard to how much input a student can have on the specifics of the curriculum. Each university also has its own philosophy as to whether part of the training can be undertaken in an environment that is not directly supervised by faculty members of the home university. Universities do have to meet accreditation standards, so while there is some room for flexibility, minimal requirements and objectives do have to be achieved.

During the latter years of medical school, you will take on significant clinical roles and may be referred to by such titles as clinical clerk, student intern, or medical student intern. It is often during these clinical years of medical school that you will begin to get a true feeling of what medicine is all about.

While most medical schools have one teaching site for the bulk of the training of the entire group of students, some schools have adopted a distributed curriculum, whereby teaching and clinical experience is offered at more than one geographic site. Some sites are limited to one specific element of the curriculum; others might provide a full-service educational experience. Some universities have a separate campus in a rural area so that students can have this type of experience. Physicians are often needed in rural areas, so exposing medical students to a rural practice during the training phase may stimulate a student to consider a career in a rural or remote location.

In North America there is an accrediting body that regularly examines medical schools to ensure that the highest standards are met. An external team of assessors visits the schools and thoroughly reviews all aspects of the programs. Medical schools also undergo self-assessment assignments and internal reviews to make sure standards are maintained and accreditation is upheld. Medical students and residents are often asked for their opinions during a review, so while in medical school, you might have an opportunity to voice your opinions, both positive and negative, to the external reviewers.

Because medical school is such an intense academic, clinical, and life experience, you will need to devote a significant portion of time to studying. You have to be prepared for missing evenings out or weekends spent with friends because you have to study, and this may even cause you to question your decision about going through medical school in the first place. You may go through a time when you feel disillusioned and even consider giving up. These insecurities are common—just ask your fellow students. Camaraderie among medical students provides some reassurance and comfort. You may feel overwhelmed during the early years, when there is little clinical exposure and excessive academic overload, or you may feel it later, when you are exposed to the realities of clinical medicine. You may worry about being asked to leave the program because you can't keep up with your peers. Remember, though, that it is rarely necessary for a medical student to be dismissed from a program for poor academic performance. (Quite honestly, some students do need to repeat a year, but rarely have I seen dismissal.)

Different teaching models are used for medical school. Some schools favor large-class instruction, while others use smaller groups. The problem-based learning (PBL) concept, for example, is a small-group learning environment. Students address a topic with the help of a moderator, who serves as a facilitator. This stimulates the students to research the topic and optimize the self-directed learning technique and group effort; the students essentially learn from each other. The facilitator makes sure things stay on track and that a weekly task is appropriately completed. Frequently, completing the task involves a number of sessions. A weekly topic is presented, and the students then have an opportunity to research the topic between sessions. They discuss it further at the sessions and finally, they arrive at a diagnosis and treatment plan.

Medical school curriculum covers an enormous amount of knowledge. In your early years, you'll take basic science courses such as anatomy and histology. The clinical aspect of medicine covers body systems—cardiovascular, pulmonary, renal, blood and lymphatic, musculoskeletal, brain and behavior, growth and development, and reproduction. As you enter the clinical years, you will encounter all the different disciplines—general medicine, surgery, pediatrics, psychiatry, and emergency medicine, to name a few. The curriculum also covers areas that are important for the practice of medicine, such as ethics, prevention, and evidence-based medicine.

One of the many advantages of our high-tech age is that a medical school syllabus is often available in an electronic format. Lectures may include PowerPoint presentations and are frequently available on Web sites for the students to review. Textbooks and journals are also readily available online. There may be a technical component of training that includes the use of simulation techniques and models for such things as resuscitation, intravenous insertion, suturing, intubations, and surgical techniques. Mannequins used in such simulation models are very realistic.

Histology may be taught using conventional slides and microscopes or with images displayed on monitors. The teaching of clinical procedures also makes use of the latest technology, such as having a monitor from an operating room show a close-up view of a procedure—the added advantage here is that it prevents overcrowding in the operating room, and the entire class is able to view a procedure at the same time. With the invention of robotic surgery and the likelihood of its increased use in the future, the face of surgical training is changing. High-tech advancements, however, are not likely to take the place of a skilled surgeon.

The opportunity to dissect cadavers varies from school to school. Some medical schools have an in-depth program that includes complete dissection of the cadaver from head to toe. Others might have limited dissection, or they may have predissected specimens that expose all the relevant anatomy. Ultimately, you will need to understand the anatomy of the human, and some schools consider using comprehensive dissection of cadavers to be the best way to impart this information.

Examinations in medical school may be oral; paper-based, consisting of multiple-choice questions, short questions, or essay questions; or computer-based, as is the format for the newly transformed MCAT exam. Another testing scenario involves the Objective Structured Clinical Exam

(OSCE), which is used frequently, particularly in the clinical years. When you take an OSCE, you will go through a number of stations that consist of different questions or scenarios, each covering a wide range of topics or questions. The stations may be written questions, oral questions, or scenarios involving specimens, diagrams, photos, video clips, and patients (actually, someone may be trained to act as a patient with a certain condition if a real patient is not available).

Medical school requires you to work together with your fellow students for long periods of time, often in small groups. During this challenging time, lifelong friendships can be cultivated, as bonding with fellow students who are experiencing the same situation makes the friendships that much stronger. Although the training is intense, it is possible to maintain a good diet, healthy sleeping patterns, sufficient physical activity, and a limited social life. Juggling a variety of activities simply requires time management and setting priorities.

From reading to note taking to talking out loud, your style of studying is your own. When I was a young medical student, I found that the more mature students were better at processing the necessary knowledge in the shortest amount of time. They often had a spouse, children, and many commitments, so they seemed to spend less time staring into space while working and they appeared to cover the material in half the time that it took the rest of us. I learned from these mature students, particularly in terms of time management and setting priorities. Some students prefer studying in study groups. This might be especially helpful for you if you have problems spending prolonged times studying on your own and maintaining concentration. Regardless of your study habits, however, I cannot stress enough that everything possible should be done to ensure you have enough time for physical exercise, relaxation, and maintaining a healthy diet. This is particularly important because as a medical student, you will frequently be exposed to viruses and other infectious illnesses. You need to keep your immune system strong with regular exercise, an appropriate amount of sleep, and a healthy diet. Additionally, your medical school will require certain immunizations. Generally, this includes immunization against hepatitis A and hepatitis B; other requirements could include immunizations against diphtheria, tetanus, and pertussis (whooping cough), and screening for tuberculosis. Blood testing for HIV and hepatitis C prior to entering medical school is a controversial topic, but this also may be required.

Learning to act with professionalism is a significant aspect of medical school. Such issues as appropriate dress, language, interaction with patients, and interaction with fellow medical staff are discussed and debated extensively. While there are no universal professionalism standards, medical schools generally have their own set of acceptable standards and guidelines for appropriate behavior, and such standards and guidelines are expected to apply to all students, regardless of one's country of origin or cultural beliefs.

No student needs to feel isolated when going through medical school. Recognizing that medical students need varying degrees of help and support, most medical schools have support systems in place. These often include the student affairs office, faculty members, staff members, mentor programs, and confidential counseling services. Student affairs staff is available for confidential counseling and are seen as advocates for the medical student body. Mentoring is beneficial for all students, so a mentor—for example, an academic, clinician, or senior medical student—likely will be assigned to help and guide you throughout the program and often beyond.

Attending medical school is an exciting, meaningful, and memorable time. There is no question that it's tough, but the knowledge and experience gained, as well as the friendships born of this time, will last a lifetime.

# 7

## *Options after Medical School*

Once you've graduated from medical school, your options are extensive. At this time, you can choose whatever route you would like to follow, and this can be modified to some degree as things progress. You may have already decided which specific area of medicine you would like to pursue, but you may ultimately practice in a completely different discipline than you once thought you would end up in. Or, you may know for certain that you've chosen wisely in becoming a doctor, but you're not sure yet whether you want to be a generalist, specialist, researcher, or academic. While it is best to pursue a specialty route once your mind is made up, if you are uncertain, there is no need to rush to make an immediate decision on your specific path. Some people wait until they have experienced as many areas of medicine as possible, as such experience aids the decision process.

Keep in mind, however, that some specialties are more competitive than others—and this can be a double-edged sword. To get into these specialties, you might have to arrange for clinical experience and elective time early on in medical school. Making a decision early on, however, can be quite limiting, as you will have made up your mind to follow a specific direction before having the opportunity to gain experience in different areas of medicine. Some examples of specialties that are generally more competitive include fields such as plastic surgery, otolaryngology, ophthalmology, dermatology, and cardiology. Generally, there are a limited number of training positions available in these specialties as compared to specialties such as pediatrics and internal medicine, where many more training positions are available.

In North America, the term "residency" is used to describe the additional time spent training to achieve the competency in the area of medicine of your choice. In the past, the term "internship" was used more frequently to describe the one-year period after completion of medical school, and this term is still used in some situations. But the term residency (or being a resident) refers to a period of two years or more, after the completion of medical school training, either to become a family physician specialist, a medical specialist, or a surgical specialist. Different parts of the world use different terminology for this post–medical school training. In the United Kingdom, for example, post–medical school training uses the terms "house officer" or "registrar." The United Kingdom also has a program known as the Foundations Program, which normally lasts for five years after the completion of medical school, in which doctors receive their primary medical qualification. The Foundations Program is a new initiative which has only recently been instituted.

You have the option to choose from numerous specialties after completing medical school. Family practice is the fastest option, as it usually requires participation in a two-year residency program. However, this does not mean it is the easiest. On the contrary, this specialty is so vast that you will be expected to have a wide spectrum of medical knowledge. Also, this training time may be extended, depending on your interest and desires. There is an option to further develop a specific skill or specialty within family medicine. An extra year or more of formal training can provide a family physician with additional skills. The family practice doctor has an opportunity to become competent in areas such as anesthesiology, obstetrics, emergency medicine, and sports medicine. Less-formal training may include interests such as psychosocial counseling, nutrition, and weight loss.

If you decide on a specialty other than family medicine, the duration of training can vary from four to eight years or more. Examples of residency programs include pediatrics, internal medicine, general surgery, radiology, pathology, cardiac surgery, plastic surgery, anesthesiology, radiation oncology, and cardiology. Not all universities or medical schools offer residencies in all fields. Some institutions are simply too small and do not have the necessary teaching staff or patient volume to offer a residency in every program. In addition, there are strict guidelines and governing bodies that regulate an institution's ability to maintain a training program.

After you've completed your residency, you may choose additional training in a subspecialty area. In North America, this is referred to as a fellowship. A fellowship lasts an additional one to three years after a residency is complete. This training can be clinical, research based, or a combination of both. Tertiary medical institutions often require the completion of a fellowship before a doctor will be considered for employment at that hospital. For example, you may become a pediatrician and then decide you would like to specialize in children's heart conditions. You can complete a two-or three-year pediatric cardiology fellowship and receive the title of pediatric cardiologist. Another example would be pediatric general surgery. In this situation, you would have to complete an extra two to three years' training after basic general surgery in order to gain the expertise needed for this type of surgery.

In many parts of North America, you will not be issued an unrestricted license to practice medicine until you complete your residency. This stipulation carries with it several implications, the most important of which is that despite being an MD, you are not qualified to practice medicine independently—not until after you complete your specialty training. This stipulation also imposes limitations on moonlighting—this refers to residents in training who wish to work after hours or in their spare time. For example, you might be a medical resident who works as a clinical assistant in an intensive care unit on a weekend day or evening, or you might be a surgical resident who works as a surgical assistant in the operating room after hours. It is important to note that moonlighting is accepted at some institutions, considered controversial at others, and prohibited entirely by some programs or hospitals.

Residency is an exciting learning opportunity, but at the same time, it can be very intense and stressful. Many jurisdictions have adopted maximum hours that a resident can work without a break, as the likelihood for error increases when one is awake for an extended period of time. A resident must stop taking care of patients after working the maximum hours of permitted. However, there are additional implications in this restriction. In the past, residents who worked extensive hours gained far more experience as they had exposure to higher caseloads and more procedures. As a result, some residency programs globally are talking about increasing the number of years of residency training in order to compensate for this shortfall. Resident bodies, associations, and unions work to ensure that the residents' training time allows for maximum learning experience, while keeping patient safety and the residents' well-being in mind.

There are also administrative bodies in place to ensure that equity is maintained in a program, regardless of age, gender, ethnic background, sexual orientation, religion, or socioeconomic status. A dean of equity might step in, for example, if a resident or student is being discriminated against for choosing to take maternity or paternity leave. In another example, the dean of equity might step in if someone is being discriminated against because of mental illness or health-related problems.

Upon successful completion of medical school in North America, the MD degree is awarded. However, it is interesting to note that *MD* is not a designation that is used universally. In many other parts of the world, including countries such as the United Kingdom, Australia, New Zealand, and South Africa, a medical doctor is given a bachelor's degree in medicine and surgery. The doctor will thus have a title such as *MB, MBCHB, MBBCH,* or *MBBS.* In these countries an MD is an additional graduate designation after the basic medical degree.

Each country has unique designations, and thus there are no standard universal certification credentials. After completing the required specialty training and certification exams, there are many additional designations possible. Examples of such titles include Fellow of the Royal College of Physicians (FRCP), Fellow of the Royal College of Surgeons (FRCS), Canadian College of Family Physicians (CCFP), Fellow of the American Academy of Pediatricians (FAAP), and Fellow of the American College of Surgeons (FACS). In the United Kingdom, as well as several other countries, a surgeon or surgical consultant might no longer use the "Dr." designation any more. These doctors are referred to as "Mr.," "Mrs.," "Miss," or "Ms." This is certainly a foreign concept in North America, and this illustrates how things can differ from one country to the next.

Obtaining that MD is only the beginning of a very exciting time. Despite the location of your training, there are many options available to you once you complete your basic medical training.

# 8

## *Specialty Options*

The scope of medicine is quite broad. The most common residencies and fellowships are listed below, but keep in mind that these are not the only specialties available.

### Allergy and immunology
These specialties are often linked, both from a training perspective and scope of practice. These doctors may choose to practice in a specific area, such as diagnosis and treatment of allergic disorders, or they may choose to limit their practice to immunological disorders. They may even limit their practice to a specific condition, such as AIDS. (Many diseases are associated with immunological disturbances.) Those who favor working with allergies spend a fair amount of time performing or supervising diagnostic procedures, such as allergy testing.

### Anesthesiology
Anesthesiology involves much more than just putting patients "to sleep." Anesthesiologists provide life support, induce memory loss for a limited period of time during a procedure, and provide pain control for surgical procedures and childbirth. In addition, they take care of critically ill patients and are actively involved in the assessment and management of patients with both acute and chronic pain.

### Cardiac surgery

Cardiac surgeons operate on the heart and related structures. Procedures can include open-heart surgery, bypass surgery, valve replacement surgery, and congenital heart repair. While this area of surgery is very exciting, some might consider it one of the more stressful fields due to the high risk related to the surgery and the related complications.

### Cardiology

This specialist deals with the heart and conditions relating to the heart. Cardiologists can choose whether or not to perform procedures. Those who perform procedures such as catheterization (inserting a catheter in the heart via distant blood vessels for diagnostic purposes) are known as interventional cardiologists. They also carry out such interventions as opening clogged heart vessels or inserting prosthetics such as a stent (an appliance used to keep a vessel open). Cardiologists are often involved with the acute care of patients in a hospital; this includes being a key member of the intensive care unit. A cardiologist also commonly deals with suspected or proven heart attacks (myocardial infarctions).

### Community medicine

This branch of medicine is concerned with the health of populations. The community medicine specialist, through a multidisciplinary approach, measures the health needs of populations and develops strategies for improving health and well-being through health promotion and disease prevention. It is not uncommon for these doctors to take on leadership roles within areas of public health. For example, a community medicine specialist may be a medical officer for a specific geographic jurisdiction.

### Dermatology

Dermatology is concerned with the diagnosis and treatment of diseases of the skin, hair, and nails. The skin is the largest and most visible organ of the body, and a dermatologist is qualified to deal with a large variety of skin disorders, including skin cancer. Cosmetic dermatology has become a widely practiced area of this specialty. Some dermatologists have a specific interest in cosmetic intervention, such as skin peels, laser treatment, Botox injections, and other antiaging skin care.

**Developmental pediatrics**
These pediatricians diagnose and manage developmental problems in children, including delays in language, motor, and social milestones, as well as cognitive impairment. For example, a developmental pediatrician's patients might include children suspected of (or diagnosed with) hyperactivity or autism. This specialty, like many, is dependent on other health-care professionals, such as speech pathologists, audiologists (hearing practitioners), psychologists, and psychiatrists. Children's development may be delayed in many different ways; these specialists diagnose the problems and work with a team to help these children.

**Emergency medicine**
Emergency medicine is a relatively new specialty. In the past, general physicians, as well as different specialists, were the first line for patients arriving in an emergency room. While this may still be the case in many emergency rooms (particularly those in smaller or rural settings), many large institutions now permit only trained and certified emergency physicians to work in their ER. These doctors take care of all kinds of emergency situations. The scope of treatment may differ, depending on the availability of specialty backup and the time it takes for that backup to arrive at the hospital. This is very much a procedural area of medicine; all kinds of interventions, many lifesaving, are performed by emergency medicine specialists.

### Endocrinology and metabolism

This specialty is quite broad and encompasses a host of different conditions. It deals with conditions involving the endocrine organs, such as the thyroid gland. Hormonal disturbances are also covered by these specialists. Many metabolic disorders are part of this specialty, including diabetes. These specialists may limit their practice to one area of interest or practice in a broader sense.

### Family medicine

The term "family doctor" is one of several designations for this type of physician, depending on personal preference, the licensing authority, or the country. Family doctors are also often referred to as general practitioners or family physicians. A family doctor is, perhaps obviously, the doctor for everyone in the family—this individual tends to children and adults. A family doctor takes care of the patient as a whole, rather than focusing on a specific area or condition of the body, as with the following medical specialties.

### General internal medicine

This doctor tends specifically to adults and is known by several different names: internist, medical specialist, or internal medicine specialist. By definition, an internist is a physician who specializes in the diagnosis and medical treatment of adults. If you choose general internal medicine, after you complete your core training (and sometimes during the training), you can subspecialize in one of several areas. Some of those disciplines are listed below. In many countries, such as those in the British Commonwealth, this type of specialist is known as a physician. In North America, the term "physician" is used for all medical doctors, regardless of their specialty. A relatively new term used to refer to a physician or an internist who works in the hospital setting is a "hospitalist." A hospitalist, however, is not exclusive to the field of internal medicine.

**General pediatrics**

A general pediatrician is the general specialist for newborns, infants, children, and adolescents. These physicians can choose to work either as a primary care pediatrician or as a consultant pediatrician, or a mixture of both. There are many interests or subspecialties that a pediatrician can pursue. While some of these doctors prefer to be working in the outpatient setting, others may choose a hospital-based practice.

**General surgery**

The general surgeon does the widest range of surgeries. Abdominal procedures are a common part of the practice of the general surgeon. The range of surgeries performed often depends on the surgeon's site of practice. For example, a general surgeon might perform a lifesaving brain procedure if there is no neurosurgeon available. Or he or she might treat fractures of the limbs if an orthopedic surgeon is unavailable.

**Genetics**

The geneticist specializes in the diagnosis, risk assessment, and management of disorders caused by changes in genetic information. These may be sporadic or hereditary disorders. A geneticist deals with patients of all ages, including pregnant women with fetal abnormalities. This is a unique specialty due to the rapidly evolving knowledge in the field, as well as the fact that information shared with an individual patient often has implications for the whole family. Geneticists work closely with genetic counselors.

**Geriatrics**

This branch of medicine concerns all the aspects of health and illness relating to the elderly. As our population ages and life expectancy rises, the scope of practice and opportunities for these physicians is on the rise too. Many doctors in this specialty choose to be part of a hospital; they then are involved in the acute and chronic care of patients who are hospitalized. Other specialists may prefer working in the outpatient setting, where they may be involved in the care of patients in other institutions, such as nursing homes.

## Hematology
Hematologists deal with conditions or disorders of the blood. This specialty is usually combined with oncology, particularly in terms of training. This branch of medicine covers the clinical and laboratory investigation, diagnosis, and treatment of blood diseases and blood-forming organs (such as bone marrow). Examples of conditions that are treated by hematologists include hemophilia (a bleeding disorder) and anemia (low red blood cell count).

## Infectious diseases
This specialty deals with any type of infection, no matter its origin. These specialists often take care of the more complex infections—those with which a primary care doctor may need assistance. This field is commonly combined with other disciplines, such as microbiology or intensive care. These physicians often work in the hospital setting, but they can also be involved in other venues, such as public health or policy making.

## Intensive care
This doctor is based in an intensive care unit, where patients with some of the most severe health problems are housed and high-risk situations occur. An ICU physician takes care of a multitude of conditions, including transporting critically ill patients. It is not uncommon for an intensive care doctor to travel to a remote destination as part of a medical evacuation team or to supervise the transport team in bringing the patient to the unit. Duties for this doctor (also known as an intensivist) also include resuscitation, inserting tubes for breathing, and administration of intravenous fluid, medications, or blood products. There are several routes you

can take to eventually end up working in an ICU, for example, respirology, anesthesia, internal medicine, and general surgery.

## Microbiology
A microbiologist is a valuable member of the health-care team who often works behind the scenes. It is not uncommon for this type of physician to head up a medical laboratory. While these doctors are often found working in laboratories, they are often called to the scene when an outbreak of a disease occurs.

## Neonatology
A neonatologist specializes in newborn babies. By definition, the neonatal period extends until twenty-eight days after birth. A large part of a neonatologist's work includes taking care of high-risk patients in a neonatal intensive care unit (NICU); these babies are often premature. These specialists may tend to premature babies far beyond the twenty-eight day mark, however, as some of these babies are several months premature and stay in the unit for extended periods of time. Frequently, these specialists also administer follow-up visits on these premature babies to monitor their development, progress, and other factors, such as potential visual or hearing problems.

## Nephrology
These doctors take care of the kidneys and conditions related to the kidneys. Nephrologists also perform diagnostic procedures, such as kidney biopsies, and can be part of a team that works together in the care of a patient. For example, when a patient undergoes a kidney transplant, the nephrologist will be a valuable member in the group of physicians that take part in the management of the patient before, during, and after the surgery.

### Neurology

Neurologists diagnose and treat conditions relating to the nervous system. The scope of practice can vary from treating a patient with a headache to treating a patient with a brain tumor to treating a patient who has a weakness on one side of the body due to a stroke. Neurologists, however, do not only take care of head conditions. Many conditions throughout the body can be neurological in origin. These doctors are often part of a team that can include neurosurgeons, radiologists, and otolaryngologists.

### Neurosurgery

Neurosurgeons perform surgery on the brain and spinal column and also cover conditions of the peripheral nerves. They often work in large trauma centers, where brain injuries are frequently present. Neurosurgeons work closely with neurologists and radiation oncologists, especially when dealing with brain tumors. Neurosurgeons are often referred to as "brain surgeons."

### Obstetrics and gynecology

A specialist in this field has expertise in the female reproductive system, including pregnancy and childbirth. The obstetrics component implies pregnancy and childbirth, while the gynecology component refers to women's health and disorders of the female reproductive system. While most doctors in this field choose to be involved in both aspects of the specialty, some might limit themselves to one specific area. This specialty is regarded as a surgical specialty, as these doctors perform many surgical procedures involving both obstetrics and gynecology.

### Oncology

An oncologist deals with consultation, diagnosis, and treatment of cancer. Like the hematologist, the oncologist often performs procedures such as a bone marrow biopsy. This specialty continues to transform as our knowledge and understanding of cancer and its treatment improves. A large aspect of an oncologist's job includes providing chemotherapy treatment to cancer patients.

## Ophthalmology

An ophthalmologist or ophthalmic surgeon is specialized to diagnose and treat eye disorders; this includes performing necessary surgeries. Some of these specialists might choose to work strictly on the medical side of this field, while others prefer a primarily surgical practice. These surgeons may be office based within an acute care facility, or they may have an arrangement at another type of facility. For example, laser surgery on the eyes is a fairly common procedure these days, and some of these specialists opt to work solely in a laser facility.

## Orthopedic surgery

Orthopedic surgeons focus on the musculoskeletal system and treat conditions such as bone injuries and fractures, arthritis, and bone tumors. They deal with the bones but also with disorders of the muscles, ligaments, and nerves. Their surgical procedures often require the use of power tools, casts, and splints. They may apply casts themselves or work with other health-care professionals who are experienced in cast application.

## Otolaryngology—head and neck surgery

Another name for this specialty is ear, nose, and throat surgery. In addition to the ear, nose, and throat, these specialists take care of conditions associated with the neck and face. These surgeons can subspecialize in many different areas. For example, some acquire extra training in facial cosmetic surgery. Depending on their area of expertise or interest, most of these surgeons work in conjunction with an acute care hospital, but they may work exclusively in a smaller facility or an outpatient setting. These specialists deal with both medical and surgical conditions in children and adults.

**Pathology**
Pathology is the study of the nature of disease and its causes, processes, development, and consequences. While some might think that pathologists work only in laboratories with dead bodies, this is a misperception. This profession also includes taking a multidisciplinary approach to patient care, diagnostic procedures, research, and education. These physicians have several options for their practice including (but not limited to) conducting autopsies, examining pathological specimens, and interpreting histology slides.

**Plastic surgery**
Plastic surgeons are often considered synonymous with cosmetic surgeons, but this is a misperception. Plastic surgeons deal with many conditions and surgeries other than cosmetic surgery. Plastic surgeons are also responsible for surgeries of the hands, as well as surgery for skin cancers and burns. While some of these surgeons choose a primarily cosmetic practice, others may choose to specialize in the other areas. These surgeons generally perform all types of aesthetic surgery.

**Psychiatry**
Psychiatrists are medical specialists who deal with the medical, psychological, and social components of mental, emotional, and behavioral disorders. These doctors can order diagnostic tests, prescribe medications, practice psychotherapy, and help patients and their families cope with stress and crises. Like many other physicians, psychiatrists often work as part of a team, which could include primary care physicians, psychologists, and social workers. Phychiatrists can work in many different settings including the acute care and outpatient environment. There is some overlap between psychiatry and psychology. Psychologists, however, are not medical doctors and cannot prescribe medications, and they deal more with counseling and psychotherapy.

**Physiatry**

This relatively new medical specialty, otherwise known as physical medicine and rehabilitation, focuses on diagnosing, evaluating, and treating patients who have limited bodily function, which may be the result of disease, injury, impairment, or disability. Physiatrists cover a broad spectrum of modalities, including prosthetics (artificial limbs), orthotics (a leg brace or splint), and other durable medical equipment. A physiatrist is not the same as a physical therapist or occupational therapist, both of whom have specialized skills but are not medical doctors.

**Radiation oncology**

These physicians specialize in treating cancer with radiation therapy. A radiation oncologist uses high-energy rays to damage cancer cells and to stop them from growing and dividing. These specialists work with a team of health-care professionals, including medical oncologists, radiologists, radiation therapists, and others. This is a relatively new area of medicine and thus a fast-developing specialty.

**Radiology**

Radiologists are specially trained to read x-rays and other types of diagnostic imaging studies: ultrasounds, CT scans, magnetic resonance images (MRI), to name just a few. These specialists also perform certain procedures, including some that are high risk. An example of such a procedure is an embolization, where the radiologist plugs a vessel to prevent further bleeding. This field has seen enormous expansion in recent years, and new equipment and techniques for imaging are added frequently. Radiologists may work in a hospital setting or in a facility not associated with an acute care center.

**Respirology**
This specialty deals with the breathing passages, lungs, and related disorders. Certain clinical domains can overlap between the different specialties. For example, these doctors can tend to allergies or sleep disorders and work in an ICU, which are also shared by other specialists. These specialists often liaise with otolaryngologists, as treatment of the airway is a large function of both specialties—respirologists dealing more with the lower airway and otolaryngologists the upper airway. Respirologists also frequently work with repiratory therapists in the acute care setting. Asthma is a common condition that these specialists diagnose and treat.

**Thoracic surgery**
The thoracic surgeon is similar to the cardiac surgeon in that both forms of surgery take place in the chest. The thoracic surgeon, however, deals with chest conditions other than the heart. He or she deals with disorders of the lungs and structures that lead to the lungs. A thoracic surgeon commonly tends to patients with lung cancer. Other chest structures these surgeons operate on include the chest wall, airways, esophagus, and diaphragm.

**Urology**
These specialists diagnose and treat conditions of the genital-urinary tract. The procedural aspect of urology can range from inserting scopes into the bladder (cystoscopy) to advanced surgery for a cancer of the urinary tract. The prostate gland, which is only present in males, and conditions of this gland fall under the umbrella of this specialty.

**Vascular surgery**
A vascular surgeon primarily performs surgery of blood vessels, including surgery of the arterial, venous, and lymphatic systems. A vascular surgeon deals with a range of conditions. The conditions may be minor (such as varicose veins) or major and life-threatening

(such as an enlarged aorta in the abdomen, which can potentially burst—a condition known as a ruptured aortic aneurism). Doctors in this specialty, however, do not normally deal with vessels in the heart or brain.

While this summary does not cover every specialty available, it should give you an idea of how vast the post–medical school education field has become and how wide the spectrum of specialization can be. Please keep in mind that the availability of many of these specialties and subspecialties is dependent on a variety of factors particular to your university or institution, but this enormous scope of opportunity and variety makes a career in medicine very attractive.

# 9

## *Practicing as a Doctor*

Once a medical degree has been earned and the post–medical school training is complete, you still have more decisions to make. Do you want to pursue an academic career? Would you prefer to be in a community practice environment? Do you want a hospital practice, a solo practice, a group practice, or a private practice? Do you want to work in an urban area or a rural area? Would you choose to work in another state, province, or even another country? Various factors can influence and limit where and how you work.

A family physician has many choices when it comes to choosing a location from which to work; this is a choice that a specialist is not often privileged to have. Affiliation with a hospital is not required for a family physician, although many do choose to maintain an active role with an acute care hospital or a long-term care facility. For example, family physicians can choose to work in a walk-in clinic, where hours are flexible and overhead commitments are not a burden. While this situation might be desirable to some family doctors, others may see this route as less desirable, as this situation often lacks continuity of care where you are able to follow up and see how your patients are doing due to the limited and sporadic exposure to the same patients.

Family doctors can further decide how much acute care they want for their practice. Some physicians might opt for delivering babies and tackling emergency shifts, while others might choose to run a purely outpatient-based practice. There are also ongoing opportunities for general practitioners to develop an interest in one of many other subspecialties of choice. Some examples include psychotherapy, sports medicine, legal medicine, aviation medicine, and disability or insurance claims. These physicians might also choose to become more involved in the procedural side of medicine, with interventions such as laser treatment, Botox treatments, hair transplants, and facial peels. A family physician may also choose to pursue a career in surgical assisting. This allows the physician to experience the surgical side of medicine without having the responsibility of being the primary surgeon and without being responsible for the care of the patient before and after the surgery. Some physicians choose surgical assisting as the focus of their entire work existence—they have fixed hours, no office or overhead expenses, and they work as much or as little as they like. Often, there are opportunities in hospitals and long-term care facilities for family physicians, including on-call duties and inpatient care. Family physicians (general practitioners) have enormous flexibility as to what type of practice they choose to pursue.

An anesthesiologist can have the freedom to design the type of practice and hours he or she desires. On the other hand, there are some limitations as to where an anesthesiologist can work. Anesthesia is usually performed in a hospital or alternate surgical facility, where it is practical and safe to provide this kind of service. Though there are smaller medical and dental facilities that provide anesthetic services, the community must be large enough to house a local hospital or surgical facility. Anesthesiologists, however, tend to perform shift work and therefore have an advantage when it comes to flexible working hours, conference time, holiday time, and travel time. Also, they don't usually have an office or the commitment and overhead that goes with it.

Demands for specific specialties change with time. For example, as of this writing, in Canada, there is a shortage of physicians from several disciplines, especially family doctors and anesthesiologists. But manpower dynamics and cycles can—and often do—change, so it is never a good idea to choose a career based solely on manpower needs. A specialty that was in high demand while you were going through your training may have few openings when you're ready to practice.

Most surgeons need access to a facility, such as an acute care hospital, to perform relevant operations. They usually must provide inpatient, outpatient, and emergency duties for the institution in exchange for operating privileges and dedicated surgery time in the facility. Depending on how many physicians are in the group, the responsibilities vary. If you are a surgeon practicing in a small community, for example, you may be the only surgeon available and thus frequently on call. On the other hand, if you work in a big city or a large institution there might be fifteen other surgeons, and so your on-call responsibilities would be less frequent. It's true, however, that the surgeon in a large institution likely will service more patients while on call than the solo surgeon in a small facility, who may be called out only occasionally.

It's important to realize that your options for your practice location will be limited as a surgeon who has specialized in a particular area, and these limitations will likely correspond to how specialized you've chosen to become. For example, a liver-transplant surgeon can perform this type of surgery only at highly specialized institutions, where the infrastructure and support for a procedure of this nature exists. And this may not necessarily be in your city of choice.

A dermatologist can work in any setting and does not necessarily need a hospital or acute care facility to function. Jobs for a dermatologist, however, are somewhat limited by location because appointments with a dermatologist are generally by referral only. The dermatologist's practice needs to be located in an area that is big enough to accommodate a sufficient physician referral base and has sufficient patient demand. One very attractive aspect of dermatology is that minor surgical procedures can be performed in the office setting. Also, dermatologists are not necessarily subjected to the on-call duties that doctors in other procedural specialties, such as surgery, are faced with.

Radiologists—doctors who specialize in medical imaging—need to practice in a facility that houses appropriate and up-to-date equipment and in an environment with trained technologists and technicians. As a specialist in this field, you must decide whether you want to work in a facility with a large selection of available equipment or a smaller facility with limited imaging equipment available. (Sometimes, smaller facilities have access only to basic X-ray machines.) But technological advancement has flourished in recent years, and this offers radiologists a particular advantage—they can receive images and provide reports electronically from a distant site, and they often have the option of deciphering images on their home computer.

If you choose pediatrics as your specialty, your mode of practice has several options. As a general pediatrician, you might choose to have an office-based practice. You also have the option of performing primary care pediatrics or performing consultations only. Pediatricians who limit themselves to a consultation practice accept patients by referral only and, not infrequently, see patients only on one occasion. Demand for services might dictate which mode of practice you choose to pursue. The subspecialty opportunities differ significantly, depending on which subspecialty you choose. A pediatric intensive care specialist would be required to spend some evenings in NICU or, periodically, be on call all night. You might find yourself up all night if there's a serious problem, or you might only need to offer information over the phone—it depends on the situation. On the other hand, you might choose to become a developmental pediatrician who only does office work. The possible locations for your practice will also vary considerably depending on the field of pediatrics you choose.

As was mentioned previously, pathologists are often mislabeled as doctors who work with dead bodies. (There's a common joke in the medical field: "If you don't like working with people, do pathology.") Yet this perception is wrong. Pathology is a vast and exciting field, and these specialists deal with patients, colleagues, staff members, students, residents, and fellows as part of their daily routine. The practice of pathology usually involves a position within a hospital or laboratory, and there are many opportunities available to those who pursue this specialty. Pathologists can work as state examiners, coroners, or forensic pathologists.

An emergency physician works full-time in an emergency room. In the past, there was no specific training program for this specialty, but most universities now offer a training program in emergency medicine, which usually lasts an additional five years past medical school. An emergency physician can be confronted with many different medical scenarios, some more acute than others; thus a broad training is required. Smaller hospitals and rural areas still offer opportunities for family physicians to work in an emergency department without advanced training or certification. The growing trend in North America at large facilities, however, is to permit only fully trained and certified emergency physicians to work in emergency departments. The advantage of this specialty area is that these doctors are dealing with exciting, acute care medicine, and they perform a variety of procedures. Depending on the financial arrangement, they usually do not have to commit to overhead and expenses, and this is shift work, so hours are somewhat flexible, but usually involve night shifts.

One aspect of practice, the issue of being on call, warrants further comment. This aspect of medicine is not only important, it's a way of life for most practicing physicians. The frequency and severity of on-call duties differ immensely from one setting to the next. Factors that influence on-call responsibilities include your specialty, type of practice, location of practice, number of colleagues in the call group, and the type of institution where you work. Some issues may be remedied over the phone; other calls will result in a visit to the emergency department. Additional factors are also involved with being on call, such as the nature of the facility. A teaching or university hospital might require that specific steps be followed in a specific order when a call comes in—for instance, that a specialty service made up of students, residents, fellows, and the attending staff physician be contacted. In such a scenario, it's likely that by the time the problem reaches the attending physician, it will have been resolved. On the other hand, a physician who is covering calls for a community hospital would be first in line to receive the calls, which may frequently result in a visit to the hospital. In the latter situation, depending on the size of the hospital, the calls may be less frequent.

I have witnessed many physicians undergo temporary personality changes while on call—this no doubt has something to do with having to rush to the hospital in the middle of the night or being forced to leave a family function or social event. It's understandable to those of us in the medical field, but your patient may not be so understanding. Remember to keep in mind that the important issue is that you are helping patients and potentially saving lives—this is a good motivator for dealing with on-call problems.

You may have decided that you want to practice in a particular location. If so, keep in mind that you may have to contend with other limiting factors, such as additional exams and licensing requirements unique to a specific state, province, or country. Some countries do not acknowledge any of the medical school or residency training of other countries. If you wish to relocate to another country, you must repeat medical school or find a new career. Obviously, if you train and then choose to work in the same country, this will not be an issue, but you still may have to contend with specific licensing requirements.

As a physician, you must adhere to never-ending requirements and controls, even after becoming certified. Most certification bodies require continuing medical education (CME), and this applies to all physicians. A certification body might stipulate the minimum number of hours of CME required each year, as well as the nature of this education, including attending rounds, lectures, courses, conferences, and conventions. These educational experiences usually must be documented in some form and submitted to the relevant licensing or certification body. Some organizing bodies require doctors to take competency exams every few years. A wealth of resources pertaining to CME is available online, including e-journals, study tools, and Web-based courses. Some licensing bodies permit you to take online courses to fulfill part of your CME requirements.

Just because CME is required doesn't mean it can't be enjoyable. It is often an opportunity to mingle with colleagues and get reacquainted with old friends from your medical school, residency, and fellowship. Depending on the forum of the meeting, you may be able to network with people who could help your career advancement. Commonly, CME events are held at holiday destinations, giving you the opportunity to combine learning with a minivacation. CME aboard a cruise ship is a popular choice. You are likely to already be very well acquainted with computer technology. The Internet is a valuable source of information—you likely will find many answers to pertinent questions just by typing a word or phrase into a search engine (such as Google). This actually has become a challenging part of medical practice, as patients have access to much of the same research and information as you do. Don't be surprised if a patient alerts or educates you about something you may not have heard of. While you may find this difficult to deal with during your early years of practice, as time goes by you likely will become more relaxed about this type of situation—you will realize that you don't necessarily have to know more than the patient about a certain subject; nobody—not even the physician—is expected to know everything all the time.

Potential medical students also should be aware that they may eventually face peer reviews by a licensing body and audits from a funding agency. Although most physicians pass these hurdles with flying colors, the mere experience can be intimidating and daunting. Peer review is a situation whereby a fellow physician or team of people (partially made up of people in the same area of practice as you are) reviews your office, files, and practice patterns to assure that you are practicing medicine within the realms of standard of care, thus optimizing patient safety. They will scrutinize your practice in any way they can to ensure that standards are being met. An audit may be carried out, for example, by a provincial or government funding agency that is responsible for remuneration of physicians. Many of these audits are purely random; others might be initiated by a red flag or a report to a licensing or billing authority. These agencies can search for many things, including billing for a patient that the physician did not treat, charging for procedures that weren't performed, or any other evidence of fraud. These authorities also send letters to patients, asking that they confirm that they were, indeed, seen on a specific day by a specific physician and that they received the services claimed by the physician. While this may be an alarming experience for you, the intentions behind the audit are sound. These procedures are essential for protecting the public, upholding the highest standards of care, and for preventing fraud.

By this point you may realize that the profession is not as glamorous as you may have once imagined. Still, the various rules and regulations serve to protect everyone, physician and patient alike. One negative aspect, however, is the possibility of litigation—something that is, unfortunately, becoming more common as time goes by. Litigation is especially prevalent in the

United States. It occurs more frequently with some specialties than with others; those areas that see more frequent litigation include plastic surgery, obstetrics, and some of the other surgical specialties. The frequency of litigation has resulted in high annual medical-protection premiums for physicians in certain jurisdictions. The premiums do, however, differ, depending on your medical discipline and which areas of medicine are more prone to litigation. As a physician, you can aspire to practice medicine only to the best of your ability—and hope that you are never involved in a litigation case. (It is not uncommon, however, for a physician to act as a third-party expert in a medical litigation case, such as in cases of motor vehicle accidents, insurance claims, and physical abuse situations.)

Student, resident, and physician health and well-being, both physical and mental, seems to be emphasized more now than in the recent past, and I am glad to see this happening. Students or residents usually have a designated physician whom they can contact with regard to their personal health issues. There generally are hotlines as well that a physician or physician-in-training can phone, twenty-four hours a day, should there be an urgent need for help. Seminars, courses, and lectures on topics relating to a physician's personal health are becoming a routine part of medical schools, faculties, and relevant institutions. Many doctors spend their lives taking care of patients, yet they neglect to find a family physician for themselves. Remember that doctors can incur the same physical and mental problems as anyone else, and it's important to take care of your own health.

As I hope you've come to realize, it's crucial for any individual who is thinking about pursing a career in medicine to be well informed of the positive and negative aspects of being a doctor. Once you have the information you need and are well informed on all the factors involved in being a physician, a medical career can be incredibly fulfilling.

# 10

## *Alternative Career Choices as a Doctor*

By the time you become a doctor, you likely will have decided that you enjoy what you are doing, and you will be content with your choice of career. If, however, you have become disenchanted or unhappy with your career choice in medicine, remember that there are always other options. Whether you feel the need for a change, want to reinvent yourself completely, or are looking for additional challenges, realize that a shift in your career path can be a realistic option.

Many physicians have a clinical practice in the earlier part of their careers and then later decide to become involved with education. If you choose this route, you can either combine academia with a pared-down clinical practice or become a full-time academic in a teaching institution. Often, this change of pace and direction is very rewarding, and the years of practical experience can be utilized in teaching future medical students, residents, or fellows; it can also include nurses, paramedics, or other para-medical disciplines. Doctors usually receive an academic rank with an institution when they join the faculty—commonly, instructor, lecturer, assistant professor, associate professor, or professor. The professorships are usually divided into clinical versus research positions, and the title can change accordingly (for example, assistant clinical professor). These divisions are based on whether a physician is more involved with clinical work and education and research or basic science research and less clinical involvement. Once again, these categories vary from one institution to the next.

You may choose to pursue a career in medical administration. This could be at the local level, university level, provincial level, state level, or national level. Some of these positions require previous experience; others allow a physician to start an administrative position at the entry level without much administrative experience. If you know that you are going to make a future change to administration, you may choose to attend leadership workshops and classes or obtain a degree, such as a master's in medical education or a master's in business administration.

Other areas in which you may choose to become involved in a new career include becoming part of a licensing body, medical association, medical protective body, or insurance company. And it's not entirely unheard of that physicians change from the practice of medicine to politics.

You may have an interest in the pharmaceutical industry during your clinical years and may choose to become involved with these companies. This pharmaceutical involvement can come in the form of continuing medical education for physicians, clinical trials, advisory boards, or consulting. Pharmaceutical companies do play a role in CME events, as they might sponsor or host an event for educational purposes. Generally, rules and guidelines are in place with regard to how pharmaceutical companies can interact with doctors in this forum. Positions within the pharmaceutical industry can range from doing research to being a medical director for the company. Pharmaceutical companies need input from doctors at many levels, and this opportunity allows doctors to share their expertise, which ultimately is to the benefit of the patients.

Perhaps you have decided that you want to specialize in a specific area after being a generalist or change to another specialty. If so, there are always options. There are always programs available that will allow you to proceed with this change in direction, which sometimes is referred to as a "reentry residency position." Sometimes, there may be a number of reserved positions in a training program that are designated for these reentry physicians.

Perhaps you realize that you're really cut out to be a business person. You might have started out as a clinician or academic, but you may later find a niche that allows you to make the transition to full-time business person. This could be related to a clinical entity, a medical invention, or something entirely unrelated to medicine. For example, a sleep disorder specialist might develop a sleep laboratory and become so absorbed and successful in the business side of things that clinical medicine is given up to pursue a successful business venture. Or, maybe a doctor who has an interest in weight loss decided to open one or more weight-loss centers. A venture like this can become a full-time business commitment (and often has income potential that exceeds what the doctor would have earned in medicine). As a physician, however, keep in mind that a business venture, such as in the above examples, involves a risky undertaking, and not all business ventures are successful.

While none of us expect it to happen, you may need to leave your chosen field due to an illness that affects your ability to function. For example, a doctor stricken with a disorder like multiple sclerosis, which affects motor functions and vision, may be forced to modify or completely change his present practice. He could, however, switch to another area of medicine where motor skills are not crucial—he may transition from a surgical specialty to a counseling-based practice, research, or administration. (In a worst-case scenario, a doctor may develop a disability so severe—from a stroke, for example, or injury from a motor vehicle accident—that he has no other option than to give up medicine entirely. This is why it is important to have disability insurance policies in place.) Life insurance policies are also important, just like in any other profession.

Physicians occasionally decide to become a consultant for an insurance company after some time in practice. Similarly, some doctors will give consultations for prosecutors or defense lawyers. These consultation positions usually require a fair amount of experience and knowledge as a practicing physician.

Whatever your reason for wanting a change, you needn't feel trapped in a profession or specialty in which you are not happy, particularly when there are so many options for doing something else. No matter how well you educate yourself and become informed about a career in medicine, there will always be situations that may cause you to be unhappy in your job. Remember that change can be a good thing, and medicine, being such a broad field, certainly allows for a change in career direction.

# 11

## *Other Challenges*

Regardless of the profession you ultimately pursue, there are bound to be challenges. In addition to those challenges previously mentioned, I'd like to add a few more to consider as you decide whether or not you want a career in medicine.

A big issue for prospective medical students is finances (or lack of them). Going through an undergraduate program followed by medical school and residency can result in major debt. The actual amount of funding required to complete medical school and residency depends on certain factors, such as geographic area and choice of public or private medical school. A debt of $200,000 (U.S.) can easily be incurred with medical school and residency training.

A large amount of funding, however, may be subsidized by the government. This allows for lower tuition fees. University Web sites usually provide estimates relating to cost, and they break it down into the different components. The time commitment and the intensity of the training you'll endure during medical school usually does not allow for part-time employment to supplement your income, which is why the debt incurred by medical doctors at the time of graduation is usually more than in other professions.

Some institutions offer scholarships and bursaries, but these are usually limited to a lucky few; this compensation is often reserved for individuals with high academic or nonacademic achievements. There are certainly other criteria that warrant scholarship or bursary money, so it is important to research each university in detail to learn what funds are available. In addition to academic scholarships, funding assistance is often offered by different groups, including the military. Do yourself a favor and thoroughly investigate and research all possible scholarships and bursaries.

Most institutions have resources in place to advise and direct medical students who are seeking financial help, as most students require loans of some sort. Usually, there is a selection of different types of loans available from financial institutions that are designed specifically for medical students and residents; these may be repayable at discounted rates, or interest payments may be deferred until a specified time after you completed your studies. I advise planning a budget with someone who has experience with financial matters. This will give you a good idea of how much money is required for the duration of medical school and possibly during residency. It is best to be fully informed of the major debts that will arise and all the different options that are available. The good news is that some medical schools provide a stipend for students during one or more of their clinical years. Often, this is because the student takes on more of a service role in combination with the educational aspect of schooling. Additionally, as a resident, you'll earn a decent salary, which usually increases with each subsequent year of the residency.

One area that can be quite a challenge during medical training, residency, and practice as a doctor, is the relationship one has with the pharmaceutical industry. With so much in life driven by monetary gain, we forget that pharmaceutical companies have to make a living too. Much of their success is related to physicians recommending, prescribing, or utilizing their product. This interaction with the pharmaceutical industry can begin as early as medical school, and it is something for you to keep in mind right from day one. There is always that fine line between the doctor and the pharmaceutical industry when it comes to conflicts of interest. While both the physician and the industry usually have the patients' best interests in mind, this barrier can be unintentionally crossed by either party. Fortunately, in North America and many other parts of the world there are strict guidelines, set by licensing bodies and medical associations, that regulate exactly what is permitted and what is not.

Not surprisingly, you won't really know how intense and stressful medical school actually is until you find yourself in the full swing of things. If your university is close to home and friends, school might be easier to handle—you'll have already established social networks that are intact and readily available. If you're far away from home, however, without people who can lend support, you may feel extra stress and have a sense of being very isolated. Remember that there are always university and community social and support groups available. It is to your advantage to get involved with organizations like these early on in a program.

Physical and mental health, a good diet, and sufficient sleep—you know by now that these are essential factors for all of us, particularly as medical school can change things dramatically. This is why it's so imperative for you to maintain a healthy balance. Find time for exercise—perhaps you can get a group together and motivate each other. Don't forget the importance of maintaining a healthy balance.

I probably don't need to remind you that doctors are human, and as such, they have problems like anyone else. Doctors' marriages can end in divorce; doctors can develop alcohol, drug, or gambling addictions. Adding to the stress of divorce or the insidiousness of addiction, however, is the fact that doctors often fail to seek the help they need, due to a fear of the consequences. Unfortunately, this can compromise patient safety. A patient's safety must come first, and if one of your colleagues shows evidence that he or she is placing patients at risk, it is your obligation to do something about it. If you can't convince your colleague to seek help, you have no choice but to report his or her behavior.

During medical school and residency training, you may find yourself in the process of self-diagnosis. As each body system is covered in the curriculum, you may find yourself identifying with a symptom or group of symptoms. You may be certain that you have any number of diseases or disorders when none is present. Ultimately, you'll be able to laugh at this aspect, as almost all of us who go through this training process are all guilty of this type of self-diagnosis. But although you'll eventually see the humor in the situation, at the time it may be quite stressful as you are sure you are quite ill. Just remember to accept your self-diagnosis with a grain of salt.

Starting a family can be challenging during medical school, especially if it's during the clinical years. While you may be intent in your desire for children, remember that clinical work requires your physical presence. Blocks and rotations cannot be missed, but absence is unavoidable if you take maternity or paternity leave. If this occurs, however, you possibly would need to repeat a year of schooling. It's something to consider.

Another aspect of being a doctor—one you may not have considered because you may be so focused on wanting to help people—is the potential conflict that can arise between you and a patient. Despite your best intentions, conflict may occur at any time during your career. Any situation has the ability to stimulate conflict, but the most common examples include differences in opinion about a treatment option, perceptions of arrogance, or inappropriate communication (including verbal abuse). For the patient, it is easy to end the doctor-patient relationship. For you as the doctor, however, ending the relationship is more complex. Appropriate notification is required, and you must follow a process that has been approved or endorsed by the local licensing authority before the relationship can be terminated. These situations are unpleasant; be hopeful that they do not occur frequently.

Maintaining appropriate documentation is an important issue for doctors. With the increasing rate of review processes and litigation, insufficient documentation can be detrimental to you and your practice. Because you likely will see many patients on a regular basis, you can't know which situation or which patient might arise as the subject of a query, investigation, or litigation. Because of this, you must legibly document all appropriate information for each patient you see. If a situation arises, even years after a consultation, follow-up visit, or procedure, the only way to recall the nature of the visit is to refer to comprehensive documentation. Traditionally, documentation has been handwritten; now, much of this has been replaced with electronic records.

Another challenge you may face as a doctor is the impact this career choice can have on your social life and your ability to meet people. This is of particular relevance for single physicians who live and work in small communities, where most members of the town will likely be your patients. Because you cannot develop a personal relationship with a patient that entails intimacy or sexual relations, it can be difficult to have a romantic relationship unless you have other outlets for meeting people.

While you hope it never happens to you, some physicians must occasionally face disciplinary action. Possible causes include incompetence, negligence, or sexual misconduct. Consequences can result in permanent revocation of a physician's license to practice medicine and possibly criminal charges and jail time. Other reasons for disciplinary action that lead to permanent or temporary suspension of a medical license include tampering with clinical notes and unprofessional behavior.

Although these are significant challenges, they should not discourage you from pursuing your career in medicine. It is simply important to be fully informed before making a decision about a challenging and rewarding medical career.

# 12

# *Other Careers Related to Medicine*

Several careers are similar to medicine, and it can be confusing how these professions fit in the big picture when you're trying to make a career choice.

## Osteopathic medicine

Osteopathic medicine is a field that is similar to traditional medicine. Going through osteopathic medical school is not unlike conventional medical school. The practice of the two professions is also very similar in terms of primary care medicine, prescribing medications, procedures, and surgery. Osteopathic medicine, however, tends to emphasize the interdependence of the body's systems, and it incorporates holistic medicine as part of everyday practice. Osteopaths also place a lot of emphasis on the musculoskeletal system and are able to perform spinal manipulations. This is something that is not common in conventional medical practice.

Although there are specialty options for osteopathic medicine, there are fewer opportunities and choices of training programs available as compared to the medical field. The field of osteopathic medicine is evolving, however, with more specialty and practice opportunities becoming available. Osteopaths are permitted to admit and treat patients in a hospital in the same way their MD colleagues do. They are also allowed to prescribe medications. Doctors of osteopathic medicine are not universally recognized—their practice is not recognized at all in some parts of the world—but a doctor of osteopathic medicine does need to be differentiated from a doctor of naturopathic medicine (ND) and a doctor of chiro-

81

practic (DC), who generally cannot prescribe medications and do not have the same hospital privileges as doctors of medicine and osteopaths.

## Naturopathic medicine

Naturopathic medicine is an important and common patient choice in terms of primary care. While naturopathic doctors utilize natural remedies for their patients, they examine patients similarly to primary care physicians. Students seeking entry into a naturopathic college face a competitive selection process, and the training is long and rigorous, just like medicine. Naturopathic doctors often work closely with a medical physician; some even share the same office. Many medical doctors also adopt a holistic approach to their practice. I know that I will use whatever natural methods and remedies with which I am familiar before prescribing medications and recommending surgeries for my patients. Many patients have a naturopathic doctor as well as their medical doctor. In those situations I have recommended that they visit their naturopathic doctor for input, especially when the patient is keen to exhaust all of his or her options prior to proceeding with medical or surgical treatment.

## Chiropractics

The chiropractic profession is also a competitive and exciting career path. It is a rapidly growing form of health care aimed primarily at enhancing a patient's overall health and well-being without the use of drugs or surgery. Chiropractic focuses on disorders of the musculoskeletal system and the nervous system and the effects of these disorders on general health. Chiropractic care is used most often to treat musculoskeletal complaints, including but not limited to back pain, neck pain, joint pain of the arms or legs, and headaches. Although it was once a field that was very distant from medicine, there are now many chiropractors and medical doctors who work together and share the same facilities. The medical doctors who are most likely to act as a liaison with chiropractors are orthopedic surgeons, sports medicine physicians, physiatrists (rehabilitation medicine specialists), and family physicians.

## Podiatry

Another profession close to a medical doctor is that of a doctor of podiatry (DPM). Podiatric medicine deals with the examination, diagnosis, and treatment of diseases and disorders of the human foot. Surgical procedures make up a large part of these health-care professionals' practice. Doctors in this field go through similar training to those who go through medical school. Also, once practicing, doctors in this field generally are allowed to operate and take care of patients in an acute care facility, the same hospital where medical doctors practice. They thus work closely with medical doctors, who often refer patients to them for foot care and certain procedures. Similarly, podiatric doctors refer more advanced foot ailments or medical problems out of the realm of their expertise to their medical colleagues.

## Dentistry

Dentistry is a well-known field, and most people know the basics of the profession. Dentists function in many of the same ways as other medical specialties They can perform surgery, prescribe medications, and admit patients to hospitals, providing they have the appropriate admitting privileges. Dentistry has become quite specialized; certain specialties function almost identically to medical specialties—there is a lot of overlap in terms of scope of work and responsibility. For example, an oral surgeon (also known as an oral and maxillofacial surgeon) requires several years of additional training, as well as some experience with general medicine. After completion of this specialty, these dental surgeons can operate in the same hospitals as medical surgeons and take on all the same responsibilities as a medical doctor would for the care of their patients. Some types of conditions that maxillofacial surgeons treat are exactly the same as certain medical specialties, namely, otolaryngology and plastic surgery—overlap occurs in facial fractures, facial cosmetic surgery, and cancers of the face and mouth.

## Optometry

Optometry is another profession that is allied to medicine, and optometrists often work closely with the medical profession. These professionals are referred to as doctors of optometry, and they often work in the same office or facility as their medical colleagues, where referrals between the two fields regularly occur. One area where the two professions overlap is in the evaluation of a patient for laser eye surgery. The optometrist will do a comprehensive eye examination to aid the surgeon in deciding whether the patient would be a good candidate for the surgery. Optometrists have many responsibilities relating to the eyes, including checking vision, prescribing glasses and contact lenses, and diagnosing eye diseases. They are limited, however, in their ability to prescribe medications in some jurisdictions, and they are unable to perform surgery independently. The type of physician they work most closely with is an ophthalmologist (a medical/surgical specialist of the eyes).

## Nursing

Nursing has become very specialized and provides a multitude of options for study and practice opportunities. While the field once required a shorter nonuniversity degree, many nurses these days are required to have a university degree in nursing, which is a minimum of four years' training. Additionally, many nurses go on to get graduate degrees. While traditionally a profession dominated by females, more and more males are going into nursing. Some nursing specialists are now taking on responsibilities that were given to doctors in the past; one such nursing specialist is a nurse practitioner. These nurses are able to examine and treat patients, including prescribing limited medications. Other nursing specialties where significant responsibilities are taken on by nurses include occupational health, community health, and public health. Nurses obviously work closely with physicians and can be involved with the education of both medical students and residents.

## Midwifery

The job of a midwife also overlaps significantly with the medical profession. These professionals assist women during childbirth. Most midwives also provide prenatal care for pregnant women, birth education for women and their partners, and care for mothers and newborn babies. Depending on the situation and practice philosophy, midwives may deliver babies in the home of a patient, in a clinic, or in a hospital. They work most closely with obstetricians and family doctors, both of whom perform deliveries on a regular basis. Pediatricians would likely be involved as well, particularly if there are concerns about the baby. These concerns can be prenatal or at the time of the delivery, fetal abnormalities being one example. A midwife does need the backup of a medical specialist in the event of an emergency. For example, backup would be needed if there were an urgent or unexpected need for a caesarian section or if a baby was in distress immediately after birth. Midwives, similar to nurses, can be involved with the teaching of medical students in topics relating to childbirth.

## Occupational therapy

An occupational therapist is a health-care professional who is concerned with restoring useful physical functionality following disabling accidents and illness. The goal of occupational therapy is multifactorial and aimed at assisting the patient in achieving the maximum level of independent function. The scope of patients can include people who suffer from strokes, cerebral palsy, spinal cord injuries, arthritis, head injuries, amputations, burns, and hand injuries, as well as people with visual, auditory, and speech problems. An occupational therapist will also work with children and adults with developmental disabilities. Occupational therapists can work in a hospital setting, outpatient facility, or in the community. They also work closely with physicians in terms of ultimately achieving a goal of restoring function as effectively as possible.

## Physiotherapy

A physiotherapist, also known as a physical therapist, treats injury or dysfunction with exercises and other physical treatments. Similar to occupational therapists, these professionals can optimize function in children and adults with developmental delay who might have limitation of movement or function. Physiotherapists provide care in hospitals, clinics, schools, sports facilities, and other locations. In some ways, this field could be interpreted as being similar to occupational therapy. Physiotherapists, however, deal more with movement and restoration of movement. Consider this example: A patient who has a stroke will need a team of health-care professionals to help with recovery. Part of the team can include a physiotherapist and an occupational therapist. The physiotherapist will work with a stiff leg to try to restore function and plan an exercise or stretching plan. He or she will follow the patient's progress and modify the treatment as the clinical situation changes. The occupational therapist will assess the patient in terms of ability to cope with daily tasks, such as eating. A management plan will then be instituted to obtain maximal independent function.

## Pharmacy

Almost everyone has had interaction of some sort with pharmacists. They are stationed behind the drug-dispensing counter in the pharmacy or drugstore and perform many functions relating to medications. Besides filling prescriptions and maintaining a familiarity with prescribed medications, they offer valuable advice to individuals about health and over-the-counter medications. If the individual needs additional help, pharmacists can point the patient in the right direction. Pharmacists undergo rigorous training and are qualified to answer many of the questions that are posed to them by the public. Many pharmacists choose to work in a hospital or other facility; they serve as a valuable part of the health-care team. Others stay in the academic setting, where they continue with graduate studies and research. Pharmacists often converse with physicians about prescriptions and treatment options. I frequently have phone conversations with pharmacists to ask for information and advice about new products or an alternate medication choice.

## Audiology

An audiologist is a health-care professional who is trained to evaluate hearing loss and related disorders, including testing for balance (vestibular) disorders and tinnitus (ringing in the ears). This professional also is trained to rehabilitate individuals with hearing loss and fit patients with hearing aids and related devices. Many audiologists work hand in hand with physicians in a hospital or medical facility; they most commonly work with ear, nose, and throat doctors. Others work independently and have their own establishments. With our aging population, audiology is very much a growing profession.

## Speech and language pathology

Speech and language pathologists, also known as speech therapists, often work closely with medical doctors. These health-care professionals evaluate and treat communication disorders and swallowing problems. Like audiologists, they obtain a graduate degree either at the master's level or PhD level. The scope of the disorders they assess and treat is vast and can range from a young child who is unable to speak to a senior who has had a stroke.

Other professional careers in which there is overlap with the practice of medicine include physician assistants, paramedics, psychologists, radiology technologists, and laboratory technologists. The fields mentioned in this chapter can be collaboratively referred to as health-care disciplines. The collaboration of all these health-care disciplines and the medical field is becoming more common, whether in the practice of the profession, cross-training, or educational liaison. More than ever, the different health disciplines are realizing that by working together, all parties can benefit, and the patient is at the center of these benefits.

# 13

# *The Hippocratic Oath: Things to Keep in Mind*

While considered outdated by many, some medical schools still require their new graduates to swear by the Hippocratic oath at graduation. (Some schools simply read the oath; others don't include the oath in their graduation process at all.) Traditionally, if the oath is going to be recited, it is done during a hooding ceremony when you graduate from medical school.

The oath has undergone several changes since the original version materialized. The exact origin is somewhat contested, but it's believed to have been written by Hippocrates in the fourth century BC. The original version was written in Greek, and several different versions have been proposed through the years. The most widely accepted modern-day version was developed in 1964 by Louis Lasagna, a former dean of Tufts Medical School in Boston. I think it is important to read through the modern version of the oath as you near the end of this book. It will help you understand the ethical expectations of a physician. This Louis Lasagna version has been obtained from the Association of American Physicians and Surgeons Inc. Web site (http://www.aapsonline.org/ethics/oaths.htm). It reads as follows:

I swear to fulfill, to the best of my ability and judgment, this covenant:

I will respect the hard-won scientific gains of those physicians in whose steps I walk, and gladly share such knowledge as is mine with those who are to follow;

I will apply, for the benefit of the sick, all measures which are required, avoiding those twin traps of overtreatment and therapeutic nihilism.

I will remember that there is art to medicine as well as science, and that warmth, sympathy and understanding may outweigh the surgeon's knife or the chemist's drug.

I will not be ashamed to say "I know not," nor will I fail to call in my colleagues when the skills of another are needed for a patient's recovery.

I will respect the privacy of my patients, for their problems are not disclosed to me that the world may know. Most especially must I tread with care in matters of life and death. If it is given me to save a life, all thanks. But it may also be within my power to take a life; this awesome responsibility must be faced with great humbleness and awareness of my own frailty. Above all, I must not play at God.

I will remember that I do not treat a fever chart, a cancerous growth, but a sick human being, whose illness may affect the person's family and economic stability. My responsibility includes these related problems, if I am to care adequately for the sick.

I will prevent disease whenever I can, for prevention is preferable to cure.

I will remember that I remain a member of society, with special obligations to all my fellow human beings, those sound of mind and body, as well as the infirm.

If I do not violate this oath, may I enjoy life and art, respected while I live and remembered with affection hereafter. May I always act so as to preserve the finest traditions of my calling and may I long experience the joy of healing those who seek my help.

There are several concepts that come to light from the oath that relate to the personality required to become a physician as well as the ethical responsibilities that are expected of a physician. I earlier emphasized the fundamental reasons that you should consider before going into medicine. This oath highlights the importance of compassion, understanding, warmth, and sympathy. I believe these characteristics are synonymous with being a physician. While these are obvious personality requirements for the practice of medicine, it is important to see these words within the text of the oath that many physicians swear by when graduating from medical school.

The ethical expectations of being a physician are important to understand. Many important ethical considerations are mentioned in this modern-day version of the Hippocratic oath; the first implies the sharing of knowledge. Someone had to teach doctors to be doctors, and thus it is expected of doctors to share their knowledge and help educate future physicians. Many other factors come into play when one opts to educate another—financial remuneration, time availability, and working conditions—but we have to keep in mind that it is our obligation to teach those who are training below us. This applies not only to students, residents, and fellows but also to the continuing medical education of those physicians who are already in practice.

Knowing a physician's limitations and boundaries is an important concept. It is impossible to know everything in medicine—or even in our own chosen discipline—and a physician needs to know when to ask for help. It may seem like a blow to your ego to admit you need help, but it is something that absolutely needs to be done. A doctor must always keep the patient's best interests first in mind. A simple example of this occurs on day-to-day basis each time a consultation takes place. A consultation typically occurs when one doctor seeks the expertise of another physician. Often, a consultation is simply a less-experienced doctor seeking advice from a more-experienced doctor, or one doctor requesting a second opinion.

Confidentiality is paramount; it is expected from and required of any physician. Patients approach their doctors with personal problems, and they need to feel secure and confident that these physicians can be trusted. Breaches of confidentiality can have serious implications for the physician, including disciplinary action and potential litigation. There are rare exceptions to this rule, such as if someone's life is in danger, but for the most part, a patient's trust in you must not be violated. This is sometimes a tough concept for a physician to abide by. You may experience challenges with a certain patient or come across an interesting patient from a clinical standpoint, and you may be tempted to mention your encounter to others. But it's imperative to learn to contain the desire to share information that would breach confidentiality.

It is not uncommon, however, for physicians to ask an opinion from another colleague when advice is needed, but there are limitations in this regard. When an informal consultation of this nature is needed, no names or identifying information should be shared. (Making an official referral for a consultation is another story; the two physicians are fully aware of the details related to the patient, including identifying information.)

An important concept highlighted in the Hippocratic oath pertains to the responsibility of a physician to see the patient as a person and not just as an illness or a condition. I really like the phrase, "I do not treat a fever chart." This quote vividly and succinctly reflects how a patient should be respected as a person and not treated as an object. In modern-day medicine, when so much of patient care revolves around high-tech investigations, advanced imaging, and electronic notes and results, we, as doctors, must remember that there is a patient behind all of this.

Prevention is as active as ever in modern-day medicine. Not only do we have health-care professionals who concentrate on the preventive aspects of medicine, but many physicians also dedicate a large part of their practice to this purpose. You may be familiar with the old saying, "Prevention is better than cure." I use this phrase frequently when assessing and treating patients. As a physician, you must be open to alternative or preventive medicines in order to optimize the health of your patients.

The word "humble" is also mentioned in this oath. It is important for you to conduct yourself in this profession without a sense of entitlement. Nobody is entitled to be a doctor; it should be considered a privilege. It is important to be modest in what you do, particularly when it comes to helping patients. Always disregard your own secondary gains, whatever they might be, and keep the best interests of the patient in mind. Don't try to prove anything to anyone for whatever reason—this relates to my original premise for going into medicine: having an unconditional desire to help people without ulterior motives of secondary gains.

As I recently reread the oath, I was pleased to see the phrase, "May I long experience the joy of healing those who seek my help." This phrase illustrates one of my main reasons for writing this book: I know too many doctors who no longer find joy in this profession, and it is really sad to see. It is my hope that if you are well informed and understand the different aspects of this wonderful profession, you will become a doctor who will have a long and joyful experience.

# 14

## *The Satisfaction of a Career in Medicine*

As you consider a career in medicine, remember to take a good look at the big picture and put things into perspective. When I reflect on my experiences as a doctor, I always think of the patients I have encountered. These encounters remind me why I am in this profession in the first place, and I'm reminded once again of how special and unique a career this can be. I'd like to relate a few of these encounters (keeping patient confidentiality in mind, of course). By sharing these experiences, I hope to provide you with an understanding of exactly why I have enjoyed much of my journey.

In family practice, a doctor sees a wide variety of patients from different backgrounds, and each has different complaints and medical conditions. Early in my career I found myself filling in for physicians who were on vacation or a leave of absence, and I tended to several small communities in a rural setting. Sometimes these small communities had only one doctor, and he or she was responsible for the medical care of all the locals. The small community hospital to which I was assigned on one occasion had three doctors. This particular weekend I was on call, and the other two physicians were out of town. One night, quite late, my pager went off—there had been a serious motor vehicle accident. Three people were hurt; two of them had only minor injuries, but the third person had severe, multiple injuries that involved many body systems.

I had recently finished medical school and postgraduate training, but no matter how well trained I thought I was, it was still a stressful and scary situation. I had no backup—I was alone and faced with a critically injured patient who was covered in blood and had bones sticking out of his skin. I knew that if I did not act quickly and keep my cool, this patient would die right before my eyes. I focused on all the things I had learned and experienced during my training. I methodically went through all the emergency skills and drills I was taught. It was my goal to stabilize this patient and have him immediately airlifted to the closest trauma center, which was about 150 miles away. Unfortunately, there was bad weather, with excess fog accumulation. This eliminated the option of a medical evacuation via helicopter or airplane and made the situation even more challenging.

Once stable, I had to accompany the patient on a three-hour ambulance ride, where further complications could occur along the way. I worked hard, with the help of the nurses, to do everything I could to get this patient stable enough so that we could make the ambulance ride. I was also in frequent contact with the experts at the trauma center. They helped guide me through some difficult procedures—procedures that weren't taught in medical school or family practice training. Thus, I was performing these procedures for the first time, but as far as I was concerned, I had no other option—it was attempt the intervention or watch the patient die. With much sweat, endurance, and time, I was able to escort this patient by ambulance on the long ride to the trauma center. It was not a relaxing trip. I had to frequently intervene to tend to low blood pressure and poor oxygen levels. I will never forget this intense and stressful ride. I wondered constantly all along the way whether or not the patient would survive.

Despite the circumstances, the patient arrived at the trauma hospital alive and in reasonable condition. Once I handed the patient over to the attending staff at the trauma center, I was free to return home. (I did hang around the emergency department until I was sure all was okay.) I will never forget the sense of accomplishment I felt, knowing I had managed to get this patient to the trauma center while he was still alive. He was further treated in the emergency department and then taken to the operating room for several procedures. I followed up on his progress, and he did reasonably well. Although I would wonder briefly over the years—during stressful times—why I became a doctor, I only needed to remember that sense of joy I felt in saving someone's life. This experience confirmed for me the reasons I'd gone into medicine in the first place.

On another occasion, I was working as part of a pediatric medical evacuation team, flying to isolated places to airlift critically ill patients to a large hospital that was equipped and staffed to handle the most complicated of pediatric conditions. A call came in that a small child, who had developed severe asthma, was having difficulty breathing. Despite all the measures the local doctor took, the child's condition continued to deteriorate, and his outlook looked dismal. My colleagues and I were in frequent communication with this isolated physician, and we knew he was not a pediatric specialist. We decided to stabilize the patient on site and then airlift him back to the children's hospital.

On arrival, we observed that the child was in a bad clinical situation; the parents were very emotional, and the attending physician was stressed and afraid. The child needed multiple specialized interventions to help him breathe and to make it safe for him to fly without further deterioration. These interventions were done under time-sensitive conditions, as every minute that went by was potentially the last for this patient. With rapid and aggressive medical intervention the patient's condition improved to a degree that made it possible to attempt an airlift without further jeopardizing his medical condition. The patient arrived at the pediatric intensive care unit in stable (yet serious) condition. His condition slowly improved over the next few days.

The amount of satisfaction and accomplishment I felt with this case was apparent on several levels. First, it is hard to describe the feeling I got from having a role in saving a child's life. The joy is almost indescribable. Next, I was able to see the parents go from such an emotional and fearful state to one of relief and appreciation—that feeling also is not easily described. Last but not least, being able to assist a fellow colleague who did not have the same expertise or experience in my field as I did also gave me great satisfaction. It was good to see this doctor, a man who initially feared the worst, regain his composure. He also played a big role in the patient's positive outcome. And he was able to go to bed that night knowing that his initial intervention and his wisdom to ask for help played a big role in the survival of this patient.

In my work as an ear, nose, and throat specialist, I frequently encounter situations similar to the last story I want to share. I often see children who have recurrent ear infections. The pain and distress caused by these infections can be quite severe, and parents are often up all night with a child who is screaming in pain. This can be an ongoing problem for months or even years. One of the ways to deal with this, if the situation warrants it medically, is to perform a minor surgical procedure that involves inserting a small ventilating tube into the eardrum. This affords an opportunity to drain the middle ear and provide ventilation to that region. While this procedure usually takes less than ten minutes and only requires a brief general anesthetic, it provides major benefits. In most situations, after the surgery, the child is free of infections. As an added perk, the parents are visibly relieved and grateful for the improvement in their child's quality of life. Situations such as these are how I know for certain that I made the right career choice.

A feeling of accomplishment is not limited to clinical areas; it also is felt in areas such as education, research, and administration. During my early years of research, I worked on mice in order to test a specific medication that was to be used after organ transplantation. I performed procedures on these mice and then treated them with a medication that suppressed their immune response. The project was stimulating in all aspects, including the microscopic surgery done on these small creatures, treating them with the medication, monitoring their progress, and finally gathering the data. After the project was complete, it was satisfying to see my published data taken into account in further studies being carried out by other individuals on different research models, namely, dogs and then humans. My research was also referenced in other researchers' articles. It was gratifying to see my name on a publication that I knew was going to be read by physicians and researchers worldwide. This is not the same kind of satisfaction I felt in the clinical scenarios, but the satisfaction was no less important or gratifying.

Teaching medical students and residents is an important function of a medical school. Their education is crucial for the advancement of the medical profession. Conducting a teaching session with a group of medical students, particularly in their earlier years, when their knowledge is limited, can be very rewarding. For me, watching students as they progress and become full-fledged doctors is very satisfying. These are the doctors of the future; seeing their transition and knowing that I was a part of it makes this part of my career very special too.

Educating qualified and practicing doctors has also been one of my strong interests as a specialist. I frequently give presentations relating to my clinical area of expertise. I usually give these talks to primary care physicians, family physicians, and pediatricians. As I have worked in all of those areas, I always attempt to approach a presentation by providing information that I would have wanted to know at a particular stage. Seeing the doctors' interest and the scope of their questions after such a session is very rewarding. And of even bigger impact to me is seeing how the physicians' practice patterns change for the better as a result of these presentations.

Finally, being in administration and having input into how things are run can be very rewarding. Often, this involves sitting on committees, sub-committees, task forces, study groups, focus groups, and panels. These groups of people make important decisions about many aspects of medical education and health care in general. In my present role in admissions, I feel an enormous sense of pleasure as I help choose our future medical doctors. For me, this has been as rewarding as my clinical, research, and educational experiences.

I hope you can see that a career in medicine can be incredibly rewarding. Every physician, whatever his or her chosen interest is, has stories that relate to how this career has made a positive impact on their lives. I encourage you to speak to as many different types of physicians as you can. It will give you a good sense of how broad the experiences in medicine can be.

# Conclusion

You now should have a realistic idea of what medical school is all about and what it is like to be a medical doctor. Important factors to consider when making this crucial career decision need to include all aspects of the profession. As a potential medical school student, you'll need to consider the positive reasons for going into medicine, as well as the negative reasons for entering the field. I hope you consider all the various points I've covered that have bearing on your decision to become a doctor. As a potential medical school student, it is vital that you come face-to-face with the situations you could encounter as a doctor. I hope I have provided you with that information.

I encourage you once again to do extensive research so that you can become as informed as possible before proceeding with the medical school application process. Speak with as many people as possible about potential career choices, including family members, friends, mentors, and others who might be able to provide a new perspective on things. Try to obtain input from people in the medical field as well. Don't be shy; ask a lot of questions.

Medicine can be an exciting, challenging, and rewarding career; I personally feel privileged to be a part of this profession. It's true that it's a rough road, and you won't be able to avoid all the negatives along the way. But the bottom line, as I see it, is that if you really want to pursue a career in medicine, the negatives won't make a difference. Yes, you'll have to make sacrifices, but in the end, you'll have the career of your dreams. And there is little in life that can match the gift of helping your fellow human beings.

# About the Author

Dr. Michael Clifford Fabian (MBCHB, FRCPC, FRCSC, FACS) has a unique background, having trained and practiced in the three major areas of medicine. After practicing as a family physician, he completed a medical and surgical specialty and practiced in both pediatrics and otolaryngology (ear, nose, and throat). He is the only physician in Canada to be licensed with this combination of credentials. In addition, he has worked and trained in several provinces in Canada, practiced in rural and urban settings, and spent time in both community and academic medicine. Dr. Fabian is currently the associate dean of admissions for the MD undergraduate program in the Faculty of Medicine at the University of British Columbia. He is also a clinical assistant professor in the departments of pediatrics and surgery in the Faculty of Medicine at the University of British Columbia and is still active in clinical medicine. He has been both a medical basic science researcher and medical education researcher and has presented and published widely. Besides his experience in Canada, he is a Fellow of the American College of Surgeons and has full registration with the British Medical Council.

978-0-595-45468-6
0-595-45468-2